Yogalands

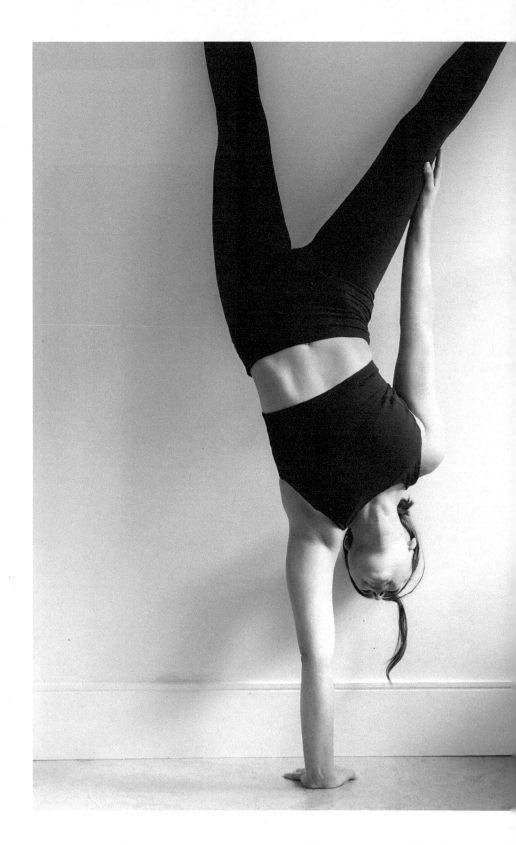

Yogalands

In Search of Practice on the Mat and in the World

PAUL BRAMADAT

McGill-Queen's University Press
Montreal & Kingston • London • Chicago

ISBN 978-0-2280-2374-6 (paper)
ISBN 978-0-2280-2443-9 (ePDF)
ISBN 978-0-2280-2444-6 (ePUB)

Legal deposit second quarter 2025
Bibliothèque nationale du Québec

Printed in Canada on acid-free paper that is 100% ancient forest free
(100% post-consumer recycled), processed chlorine free

This book has been published with the help of a grant from the Federation for
the Humanities and Social Sciences, through the Awards to Scholarly Publica-
tions Program, using funds provided by the Social Sciences and Humanities
Research Council of Canada.

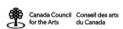

We acknowledge the support of the Canada Council for the Arts.
Nous remercions le Conseil des arts du Canada de son soutien.

McGill-Queen's University Press in Montreal is on land which long served as
a site of meeting and exchange amongst Indigenous Peoples, including the
Haudenosaunee and Anishinabeg nations. In Kingston it is situated on the
territory of the Haudenosaunee and Anishinaabek. We acknowledge and thank
the diverse Indigenous Peoples whose footsteps have marked these territories
on which peoples of the world now gather.

Library and Archives Canada Cataloguing in Publication

Title: Yogalands : in search of practice on the mat and in the world /
   Paul Bramadat.
Names: Bramadat, Paul, 1967- author
Description: Includes bibliographical references and index.
Identifiers: Canadiana (print) 20240491483 | Canadiana (ebook) 20240492528 |
   ISBN 9780228023746 (paper) | ISBN 9780228024439 (ePDF) | ISBN
   9780228024446 (ePUB)
Subjects: LCSH: Yoga. | LCSH: Yoga—Social aspects. | LCSH: Yoga—Thera-
   peutic use.
Classification: LCC B132.Y6 B73 2025 | DDC 181/.45—dc23

This book was designed and typeset by studio oneonone in Minion 11/15.
Copyediting by Robert Lewis.

This book is for yoga teachers who wonder what draws students to their studios, for students who are curious about the links between their bodies and the larger world, and for scholars who wonder how to remain human when they study what enchants them.

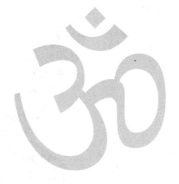

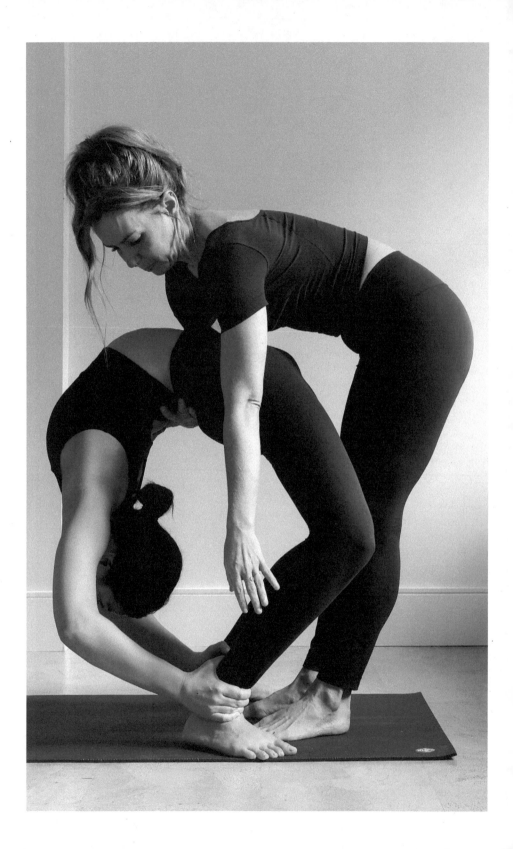

Contents

Figures

All of the figures are contemporary photographs of asanas modelled by yoga instructors Kimber Allan and Carolyn Ferreira. The photographs were taken by Molly Cameron.

FIGURES

Acknowledgments

I begin by thanking the hundreds of people who welcomed me into their classes, homes, and studios to practise and talk about yoga over the past several years. They were so sincere and passionate about understanding yoga in our society and in their lives that we often spent far more time together than either of us expected. I was humbled by their approach to the questions I posed and grateful for the ways their answers took the project in unanticipated directions.

Jeff Lichty and Rachel Reid, my first and most patient teachers, continue to clear away the smoke my mind creates. I value, and need, a lot of teaching and teachers, among whom several stand out for their sage advice and exemplary adjustments: Kimber Allan, Carolyn Ferreira (photographs of whom are featured in this book), Arielle Nash, Michele Archibald, Siobahn Sears, Rachel Mark, Harmony Slater, Angela Jamison, and Geoff Mackenzie. My body and my imagination thank you all.

Initially, I was quite worried about writing for both scholarly and general audiences. When I asked for advice from my colleagues and friends Francis Landy, Rebekka King, Patricia Lane, Rachel Brown, and a few other researchers at the Centre for Studies in Religion and Society (CSRS) at the University of Victoria, they all encouraged me just to begin the book so that I could see how it felt to adopt a more personal tone. If readers feel that I have been either too accessible or too technical, the blame lies with me. Still, I am thankful to those who understood correctly that I was indeed seeking permission to adopt an unconventional approach.

As the research assistant for this project, Leah Mernaugh (an American doctoral student at UVic) helped me to travel an enormous distance, both physically and conceptually, before, during, and after our intensive fieldwork. She coordinated interviews, class times, site visits, special events, transit routes, conference proposals, consent forms, promotions, correspondence, and focus groups. She also read chapter drafts, caught ambiguities, and asked relentlessly astute questions. When it came to our US sites, Leah's anthropological perspective was invaluable.

I am very fortunate to work with Rachel Brown, the research and program coordinator at the CSRS as well as a close colleague and friend. She was instrumental in helping me to submit the grant application that enabled the project. She also served as a research assistant for one of the fieldwork sites, which allowed me to test interpretations I was developing. During fieldwork, she was not a yoga insider (although I sense a conversion may be imminent), but as a religious studies scholar, she asked superb questions about the people we met, the places we visited, and the intuitions we both had. Having her eyes on earlier drafts of these chapters gave me some peace of mind about the direction of the book.

Several other colleagues and friends offered advice on my interpretations of what I was experiencing. My thanks to Raj Balkaran, Scott Dolff, Susie Fisher, Anya Foxen, Mar Griera, Anna Halafoff, Rosie Hancock, Andrea Jain, Pamela Klassen, Amanda Lucia, Cole Mahtani, Minelle Mahtani, Christopher Jain Miller, Géraldine Mossière, Arielle Nash, Karen Palmer, Shyam Ranganathan, Adheesh Sathaye, Jenn Selby, David Seljak, Eddie Stern, Devyani Tewari, Anna Lee White, and Katherine Young. Three generous anonymous peer reviewers also helped me to sharpen my arguments. In addition to sharing her wisdom on yogaland, Zoë Slatoff checked my translations of Sanskrit terminology. Chris Daniel Miller stepped in at the eleventh hour to offer invaluable guidance on the best way to display and interpret my survey data.

I integrated most of the advice I was offered, but sometimes I relied on instinct. In any case, any remaining errors or shortcomings are mine.

Writing this book forced me to grapple with parts of myself – what I carry, what I convey, and where I come from – that I would probably have set aside indefinitely. Facing these elements of my own story is easier when I can see them as versions of what I hear from others, such as my sisters and other nonwhite girls and women or boys and men who struggle to settle the score their bodies keep in a society that seems to offer so few opportunities for healing.

ACKNOWLEDGMENTS

This book and the project that inspired it would have been impossible without the support of a grant from Canada's Social Sciences and Humanities Research Council. The Canadian intellectual landscape would look quite different without the kind of work that this funding body enables.

Several years after she left UVic, Zoé Duhaime, a former student and rising star in the literary world, casually asked what I was writing. When I sent her a few paragraphs of this book through Instagram, I had no idea it would be the beginning of an interaction that has contributed so much to the book you are holding in your hands. The scholarly critique offered by peers and reviewers is irreplaceable. But Zoé's engagement was of an entirely different sort – mostly related to the music of the text and the kind of voice I should use, whether I was offering sober observations, telling stories, or making jokes. No one has ever been so acutely attuned to dissonances and harmonies in my prose that I sometimes could not detect.

I am indebted to Kyla Madden, acquisitions editor at McGill-Queen's University Press, who was generous with her time and energy and who offered me the kind of sustained intellectual engagement, close reading, and personal enthusiasm of which authors rightly dream. Kyla and her colleagues Lisa Quinn, Kathleen Fraser, Anna Del Col, Jacqui Davis, and Jennifer Roberts have been steadfast in their support. Indeed, four of them accompanied me to a yoga class in Montreal on a sweltering summer day in 2024, which must set a new standard for author-publisher cooperation. Robert Lewis provided expert copy-editing, a special skill that would surely be on a list of siddhis in any contemporary version of the *Yoga Sutras*.

Whatever else I might discover or imagine about my svadharma, it will always involve Karen Palmer and Max Bramadat. Thank you.

Glossary of Sanskrit Terms

ahimsa	nonharming
angas	limbs
apana	downward and outward energy
asana	yogic posture
atman	higher self
avidya	ignorance of reality
bhakti	theistic and devotional
bhakti yoga	path of devotion
bindu	point in the body where creation begins and is unified
brahmacharya	actions for the sake of Brahman
Brahman	ultimate reality
Brahminical	priestly
chakras	energy centres
citta vritti	endless whirlpool of thoughts or fluctuations of the mind
drishti	gaze
guru/ji	spiritual teacher
hatha	physical yoga practices (lit. "force")
jivanmuktas	superpeople (lit. "liberated while living")
jnana yoga	path of knowledge
kaivalya	solitude and liberation
Kali Yuga	age of decline
karma	cause and effect
kriyas	practices to detoxify the body
kundalini	coiled serpent of energy in the body
mala	garland of beads
moksha	liberation
nadis	energy channels

namaste	a bow to you
niyama	rules, guidelines, or observances
pada	chapter
paramaguru	preceding guru
parampara	uninterrupted succession of gurus (lit. "one following another")
prakriti	material nature
prana	inward and upward energy
pranayama	breath work
pujas	offerings
purusha	consciousness
sadhus	ascetics
samadhi	meditative absorption
samsara	cycle of birth, death, and rebirth
samskaras	patterns of thought based on memories
shakti	power, energy, or force
shala	yoga studio (lit. "home")
shishya	student
shlokas	verses
siddhas	perfected beings
siddhis	special powers
sthula	gross
sukshma	subtle
sutra	aphorism or instruction (lit. "thread")
svadharma	personal duty in the world
svadhyaya	self-study or introspection
tapas	heat
vinyasa	transition
yamas	restraints
yogavidya	science/knowledge of yoga

Yogalands

INTRODUCTION

Samasthiti

I stared up the long staircase leading to the Ashtanga yoga studio. After working for so many years to think about religion and society in an informed, critical manner, I felt deeply ambivalent. Why enter an environment where I was likely to be aggravated by a banal spirituality, the creeping tendrils of capitalism, impossible beauty standards, and the appropriation of South Asian religions?

Also, I had moved to Canada's West Coast from the Prairies about five years earlier, and I had promised myself that I would not become one of those newcomers who buys a kayak, becomes a vegan, begins a yoga practice, and uses social media to report on the joys of operating a lawnmower in February.

But here I was, gazing upward and wondering whether I *could* actually climb the entire staircase. I had visited my doctor several weeks earlier to address the excruciating pain in my knees. I had put running and soccer on hold, and for several months, it had been difficult even to walk my dogs around the block. My family doctor is very good at his job, and when he looked at my X-rays and then into his diagnostic tool kit, the prognosis was clear to him. He sighed, shook his head, and quoted from the radiologist's report. At forty-five, I had the knees of a seventy-year-old.

When I asked him whether dietary changes, massage, physiotherapy, acupuncture, or yoga might help, he rolled his eyes almost imperceptibly and shrugged his shoulders. He said that some of these interventions might offer temporary relief but added that they were quite expensive and unproven. He delivered the news in a caring but matter-of-fact manner: my osteoarthritis would require pain management and knee replacement surgery.

When I told some friends about my predicament, one recommended yoga. Ordinarily, with my doctor's, my peers', and my own misgivings in mind, I would have dismissed this possibility. I did not want to be that guy: the kayak, the yoga, the not listening to medical professionals. Nevertheless, the friend in question was a former elite athlete with an Ivy League doctorate. Not only did he swear by yoga as a means of managing his own aches and pains, but he is also one of the most no-nonsense people I know. I was desperate, so I agreed to try a single class at the studio he recommended. I had very low expectations.

One Saturday morning in November 2013, I hobbled up the many stairs of the Ashtanga yoga studio to attend a class, and everything changed. The transformation was not immediate. This is not a Road to Damascus story, but it is – I see more clearly as I retell it – a conversion story nonetheless.

A few years later, I did buy a kayak, but that is another story.

To be clear, this book is not about me. Indeed, readers familiar with the academic study of, well, anything will be aware that one's personal experience always threatens to obstruct a clear account or analysis of, well, everything. There are good reasons why any proper analysis should include, and perhaps even begin with, some skepticism about one's ability to provide a level-headed account.

For the first time in my professional life, I am not just an observer. Now I am also the object of my own gaze. Straddling the insider-outsider line comes with its own risks, of course, and so before I began I made certain promises to myself and my peers: I would not slight rival yoga "denominations," downplay sexual misconduct scandals, or endorse the medical benefits or the spiritual uniqueness about which yoga enthusiasts boast. These commitments were not difficult to honour, but I worried about the impact of more subtle biases. For academics in the social sciences and humanities, the first and most basic step toward making sure that one's "positionality" does not ruin one's thinking, writing, or teaching is to disclose it early on.

With that in mind, I should share that I have adopted a fairly traditional Mysore-style Ashtanga practice.[1] What this means is that I practise six days a week, about 90 to 120 minutes each time, beginning at around 6:00 a.m. I practise under the supervision of very advanced teachers who "give" me asanas (postures) within an established sequence, presenting them one at a time when they think that I am ready. Non-Ashtangis would recognize many of these asanas because most yoga styles in North America rely on movements and shapes systematized by the so-called father of modern postural yoga, Tirumalai Krishnamacharya, who taught Pattabhi Jois and B.K.S. Iyengar, the leaders of the influential Ashtanga and Iyengar lineages respectively.

A newcomer to an Ashtanga shala – meaning "home" and commonly used instead of studio[2] – would enter the room and see people practising asanas on their own, with occasional input and hands-on adjustments from one or two teachers. In fact, each student is moving through a sequence of postures that has been practised in more or less the same manner for nearly a hundred years (more on that controversy later). Since each student arrives at the shala at different times, has reached a different stage in their practice, and faces different bodily challenges, novices in the "Mysore room" are often disoriented. A student who is not yet able to touch their toes and is learning the first few standing postures will look to their side during adho mukha shvanasana (downward-facing dog pose; see figure I.1) and witness the student next to them moving effortlessly through tittibhasana B (firefly pose B; see figure I.2), a standing posture in which one folds forward and moves the torso through the knees such that the backs of the shoulders rest on the calves, and then the student binds their hands behind their back, at which point they duck-walk five steps forward and five steps backward.

When I first saw this difficult posture, I looked around to see whether other people were gawking too. When no one seemed to be even slightly curious, I whispered, mostly to myself, "Oh my God. Are you kidding?"

It may be relevant to know that my late father (d. 2004) was an Indo-Trinidadian who had immigrated to Canada in 1959 and that my mother is of Anglo-Celtic settler stock, her ancestors having come to Canada from the United Kingdom roughly three generations before she was born in 1938. A

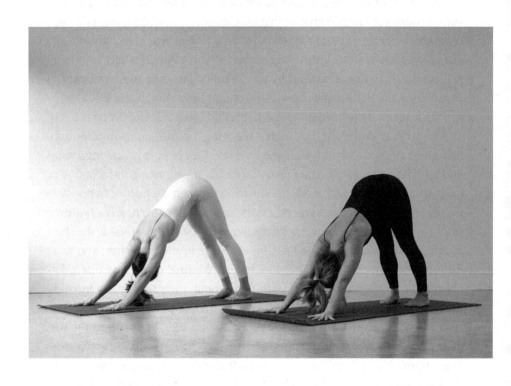

Figure I.1
Adho mukha shvanasana (downward-facing dog pose)

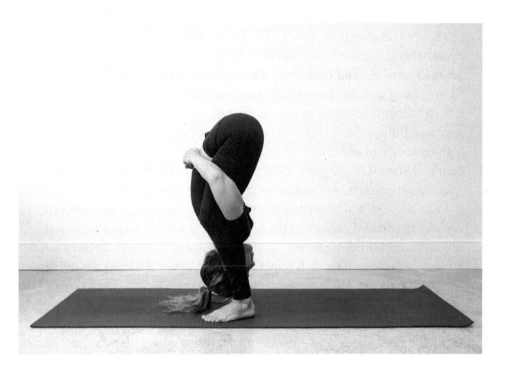

Figure I.2
Tittibhasana B (firefly pose B)

story embedded within the Indian side of my family speaks of our Brahmin origins – hence my surname, I was told. There is some evidence in support of the story told in my family about our high-caste origins, including the kinds of professions pursued and the prestige enjoyed by my male forebears – even after they converted, although briefly, to Presbyterianism, as ambitious West Indians often did to get on the right side of the colonial masters.

Before I entered my teen years, it was clear to me that my father – a school principal, champion of Canadian multiculturalism, and leader within the Caribbean Canadian community – faced formidable obstacles in Canada because of his skin colour. (My sisters and I faced our own challenges, which are too numerous and difficult to catalogue here.) I certainly understood from a young age what I know better now, namely that the caste system has caused tremendous harm to people throughout South Asian – and more narrowly, Indian – history. Nonetheless, during my youth, the story of our high-caste origins allowed me to imagine that my family had an inalienable dignity that most of my peers could neither understand (so it was a kind of spiritual superpower) nor nullify (even if some certainly tried).

I was disheartened in my late twenties to read in an article by Peter van der Veer and Steve Vertovec that the story of our Brahminical (priestly) roots might just as easily be an invention. It turns out that among indentured labourers in the late nineteenth century, there were people sometimes called boat Brahmins who left India as members of nonpriestly castes and arrived on the docks in Trinidad, Suriname, Guyana, or Jamaica many weeks later with the spiritual swagger associated with Brahmins.[3] I met Peter and Steve in my late forties when I was at a German research centre they directed. In my first meeting with these academic titans, I was about to joke that they had ruined a story that had served as a shield in my childhood, but the quip fell apart in my mind when I realized that the story had long since served its purpose: I had survived.

I am agnostic about the Brahmin roots story now, but this aspect of my biography became more resonant when I learned about Swami Vivekananda, the famous guru whose 1893 appearance in Chicago at the World's Parliament of Religions is often cited as the moment that yoga arrived in North America.[4] A few years into my own yoga practice, as I was rather casually reading about Vivekananda, I learned that he was part of religious and political reform movements in India – such as the Brahmo Samaj – that were deeply influenced *in India* by Unitarian missionaries.[5] Although the tradition has changed dramatically since the nineteenth century, Unitarians of the swami's era were still liberal Christians (mostly based in the United Kingdom and North America) whose egalitarian, rational, and universalist tendencies appealed to Hindus interested in clarifying their practices and perspectives and in promoting the universal value of their own traditions to Westerners.

To many readers, this Unitarian influence might seem like an unimportant fragment of colonial religious history, but it made me sit bolt upright because my mother had been a Unitarian minister for decades, and I had seriously considered entering this profession myself at one point. I confess with some embarrassment that when I learned about the influence of Unitarianism on some of the people most responsible for the arrival of yoga in the West and on the emergence of modern India itself, I had to resist the fleeting and clearly magical idea that my new-found passion for yoga might be part of a preordained path I was meant to walk, a revelation of my svadharma (personal duty in the world).[6]

Proper, grown-up cosmopolitans know that one of the most banal modern spiritual certainties is that "everything happens for a reason." It strikes me that when people make claims about the purposeful connectedness of all events or about what coincidences reveal to them about their svadharma, they do not often think through what it might mean for such interconnectedness to be responsible for the way the world works in general. There is nothing vicious about this common sensibility, and for all I know, it might be correct, but it does presuppose a world in which many billions of divinely ordained fates are coordinated by a cosmic event planner.

Of course, this idea is specific neither to Hinduism nor more broadly to India. It is alive and well among evangelical Christians too.[7] I appreciate the appeal of a universe that might be this orderly and a divine being who might be such an excellent choreographer, but it has never been compelling to me. So, as soon as these thoughts and feelings welled up in my consciousness, I stiffened against myself. I knew who I was, or at least who I wanted to be. Dispassionate adult curiosity needed to be my guide, even though my ego glowed brightly when I thought for a moment that my svadharma might somehow be connected to Vivekananda and, through him, to some kind of universal order.

I share my own ethnoreligious origins and details about my asana practice because they are in the soil out of which this book has emerged. I have advised graduate students and junior colleagues for many years, and I still encourage them to remember the moment in their lives when they were reading a book, visiting a temple, or washing the dishes and suddenly something seemed, well, weird, causing them to devote years to trying to make sense of it.

For me, the weird moment was finding myself in samasthiti (equal standing pose; see figure I.3) on a rented mat in Victoria, British Columbia – arguably the most British of all North American cities – hearing my fellow students join in the Sanskrit call-and-response invocation, and having a powerful sense that the previously well-separated personal, scholarly, familial, and physical dimensions of my life might be tributaries of the same river, flowing toward ...

But wait! Wait! My fingers revolt against this denouement. The same *ocean!* The same *ocean!* The same *ocean!* (Apparently, I cannot resist.)

That cluster of experiences – the invocation, the bizarre bodily shapes I see or make every morning, the temptation to enchant my own story, the way skepticism complicates even the things one feels to be most true – was certainly weird. Although these experiences were somewhat jarring at first, over the years they have allowed me to bridge or at least to measure the divide between my intimate and intellectual worlds.

At the beginning of many North American yoga classes, students are encouraged to "set an intention." In the most basic sense, what is the intention of this book? Fundamentally, I am interested in what a skeptical but devoted insider's perspective might reveal about yoga in North America. Beyond this intention, however, I am curious about what it might mean to think dispassionately about anything – not just yoga but also religions, societies, families – that one loves passionately. It seems to me that looking closely at the ways yoga is experienced in carefully situated bodies and communities – with my own body and experience being part of the data, so to speak – helps us to grasp larger crises in identity, the nation, health care, religious institutions, the climate, and the digital age.

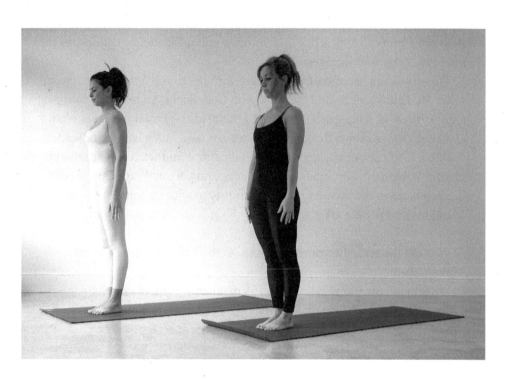

Figure I.3
Samasthiti (equal standing pose)

My focus is on students and teachers; I use the word "practitioners" to refer to both groups. I make an effort to remind readers of the many other dimensions, or "limbs," of the yoga tradition, but I am interested mainly in what the historian of yoga Elizabeth De Michelis calls "modern postural yoga,"[8] which is to say asana-emphasizing yoga, because that is almost exclusively what North Americans picture when they hear the word yoga. I spend most of my energy on the contexts in which the vast majority of North American postural yoga takes place, which is in mainstream studios, as well as in one's home, but practice there is often still informed by studio-based teachers, styles, and lineages.

There is a long list of books that begin with the title *What We Talk About When We Talk About ...* and then end with *God, Books, Anne Frank, Dumplings, Hebrew,* or some such focus. The general idea is that dumplings, God, and books are windows through which we can see a much larger landscape.

When I talk about yoga, what will I talk about and what might remain unsaid? I use stories, interviews, survey data, and personal experiences both in classes and in the broader yoga community to address some of the main questions that people ask about yoga:

- Why are the same two or three books on the bookshelves of almost every studio?
- Why do people use words – or perform an entire chant – in a language that almost no one in the room understands?
- Why do practitioners not talk much about the special powers promised in yoga texts?
- Why are about 80 per cent of North American yoga practitioners white women?
- Why do teachers in some yoga communities address students in ways that the students would never tolerate outside of class?
- How have communities responded to sexual misconduct scandals?
- How do practitioners relate to India?
- Do Canadians and Americans think about yoga in the same ways?
- How might we explain the rise of trauma-informed yoga?
- Why do teachers and students often say that asana practice is spiritual but not religious?

I will also address those features of the yoga scene that fascinate scholars of religion and society: feminism, misogyny, nationalism, authority, colonialism, charisma, attitudes toward public health and safety, and the debates over the origins of yoga. Most of the main yoga studies scholars – such as James Mallinson, Andrea Jain, Amanda Lucia, Mark Singleton, Anya Foxen, Joseph Alter, David Gordon White, and Edwin Bryant – are present either on or, more often, just below the surface of these pages. Scholars and more curious practitioners may want to consult the bibliography for suggested readings, as well as the endnotes of this book, where I try to connect readers to some of the main figures and debates in the burgeoning field of yoga studies. That is another way to say that readers should look elsewhere if they are mainly interested in Samkhya philosophy, the roots of a specific lineage, the postural yoga practised in a small number of North American Hindu temples, the dating or authorship of the *Yoga Sutras*, or the role of asana practice within bhakti yoga (the path of devotion). These issues are important but not to me, or at least not here, and there are others who are better positioned to offer learned insights about such matters.[9]

The stories that I have to tell and the context that I can provide in the chapters and endnotes might be said to concern jnana yoga (the path of knowledge) or svadhyaya (self-study or introspection) for practitioners, as well as to comprise a reasonably sober but personally informed account of complex cultural phenomena for scholars. My hope is that combining my formal academic training in the study of religion, spirituality, and society with a willingness to subject my own experiences to critical reflection might enhance our growing understanding of "yogaland," a term that I borrow from Patrick McCartney.[10]

Yogaland refers to the global yoga community, but it might also be imagined as a world or subculture just adjacent to the conventional world. People move within yogaland, whether this travel occurs virtually through podcasts, playlists, and online yoga classes or whether it involves trips to workshops, conferences, retreats, and ashrams around the world. As with all well-developed communities, certain norms and ways of talking emerge that demonstrate that these spaces are, indeed, set apart from ordinary life. However, even if yogaland promises various kinds of liberation from the limitations of normal life, it cannot entirely free itself from the nations, states, and world in which its practitioners live. Indeed, I have chosen the evocative title *Yogalands* for this book just to remind us that there are innumerable connections between the world and what I describe below as the anti-world of yoga.

The Data and Its Uses

First, however, I should say something about the research project that animates this book. After about a decade of reading and trying to contribute my small voice to the conversations around modern postural yoga, a large research grant allowed me to go out into the field in order to collect quite a deep new pool of data.

Although academics might see this book as a marriage of religious studies and critical autoethnography,[11] the truth is that I use a variety of methods and perspectives. Readers will see the way that these research elements are used to tell the story I want to tell, but let me begin by noting that during our fieldwork in seven North American cities, we conducted in-depth formal interviews with eighty-three teachers; often lengthy informal interviews with thirty-four teachers and students; twelve focus groups involving forty-three students; participant observation; and what one might call deep hanging-out.[12]

The 117 formal and informal interviews took place in homes, restaurants, coffee shops, studios, university offices, and public parks, and they lasted, on average, seventy-five to eighty minutes, with the durations ranging from forty minutes to two and a half hours. Roughly one-fifth of the teachers were also studio owners, co-owners, or managers. Initially, the open-ended interviews were designed to address several key concerns: race, health, the US and Canadian political climate(s), personal attachment to yoga, the significance of yoga as a "spiritual" practice, cultural appropriation, and the sexual misconduct controversies of the past decade in yogaland. My focus changed, but more on that later.

In theory, the project research assistant and I were able to cover these issues in roughly forty minutes, but almost all of the participants wanted to spend more time engaged in conversations that covered a great deal of territory. We met with people from a wide array of yoga traditions: Anusara, Ashtanga, Dharma Mittra, hot yoga (previously Bikram), Iyengar, Kripalu,

Kundalini, Sivananda, restorative, Yin, and what we might call nondenominational or nonlineage hatha, vinyasa, flow, or fitness-oriented forms.[13] The focus groups, with forty-three participants, involved students from a similar range of yoga styles and lasted roughly ninety minutes each. The actual identities of interview subjects are protected by pseudonyms as well as by the alteration of unimportant background details.[14]

I should note that it is arguably the case that postural yoga mostly occurs in two contexts: in communities that are not associated with a specific lineage and (especially since the COVID-19 pandemic) in practitioners' homes. But about half of the stories I tell throughout this book are set in communities associated with the more popular postural yoga brands, such as Iyengar and Ashtanga (with an emphasis on the latter), largely because these spaces provide the best canvas on which to paint a larger picture.

However, it is important not to overstate the differences between these different kinds of spaces. Nonlineage spaces by definition almost never feature references to or photos of gurus, but indirect references to lineages or at least strong allusions to Indian ideas and practices are often still there.

The most obvious example of the presence of lineages in nonlineage spaces is the sometimes quite detailed biographies associated with a studio's teaching staff. In many of these accounts, there will be allusions to a teacher's training at official Kripalu, Sivananda, or Iyengar sites, for example. There might be references to the teacher's current local mentor, the lineage affiliations of whom are either stated or not difficult to infer. Or perhaps the biography will describe a teacher's time spent in India, often with reference to lineage-identified yoga schools or cities such as Pune or Mysore, which are usually code for Iyengar and Ashtanga respectively. It is often the case that in the home settings where people practise alone, many of the teachers who are digitally or imaginatively present are themselves products of the main lineages and – whether or not it is known by the students – are teaching asana styles and sequences that emerge from these traditions.[15]

Some of the richest insights in this book came from our own bodies. Instead of just talking with teachers and students and visiting studios, my research assistant and I took classes in each of the cities that we visited. In many but not all cases, the classes were taught by teachers we interviewed or were held at the studios where they taught. It is impossible to imagine undertaking this research without also committing ourselves to spending time in these spaces and actually taking classes. During our fieldwork visits, we took a total of sixty-five classes. In some cases, we took the same class, in which case we could debrief afterward about our often quite distinct experiences. When we took different classes, we could share our impressions about the students, teachers, and styles that we encountered.

This approach meant that on sixty-five occasions, we entered unfamiliar spaces and had to figure out how to dress, behave, store our clothes and valuables, and pay for the classes, as well as when and whether it was appropriate to speak to other students and teachers. Most classes took place in yoga studios. Some took place outside, with the sheep meadow in New York's Central Park being the most memorable of these settings. Some occurred in fitness-oriented gyms such as GoodLife Fitness. A few happened in unusual environments such as a public library near the headquarters of the Self-Realization Fellowship and an art gallery a few blocks from Skid Row, both in Los Angeles. Two of my favourite classes were led by the legendary Ashtanga teacher Eddie Stern at the famous Broome Street Temple in the SoHo district of Manhattan.

Of course, although learning about this or that teacher, style of yoga, or community by taking asana classes in situ was indispensable, an equally valuable aspect of visiting these cities was that we had to travel to and navigate our way around places with which we were often only vaguely familiar, which would not have been the case if we had conducted the research strictly through Zoom or surveys. During the past few decades, I had spent time in the seven cities, but visiting these places for this project changed my experience significantly.[16] By meeting so many locals and by travelling around so much, we saw that each city had its own geography, climate, social problems, beauty, history, and for lack of a better word, vibe. These facts clearly had an impact on the yoga and yogis we encountered.

In addition to these qualitative forms of data, I conducted an online survey of 650 yoga students and teachers from all over the United States and Canada, which strengthened our capacity to reflect critically on postural yoga. I have woven survey results into the stories that I tell in this book and in the endnotes.[17]

I paired US and Canadian cities to allow us to make sensible contrasts. New York and Toronto are paired as the big eastern cities in the project. Both of them are much-storied in their larger national contexts, being reviled, affluent, beloved, crowded, complicated metropolitan and multicultural spaces. Winnipeg and Indianapolis are paired as the mid-western prairie spaces with some similar demographic and political features and with perhaps similar roles in their respective broader national stories as scruffy, often overlooked, highly racialized cities that are also unpretentious and rich in culture and history. And finally, Vancouver and Los Angeles constitute the obvious West Coast pairing, as both have not only been central players in the arrival and acculturation of postural yoga in the rest of the country but are also well known for a laid-back, you-do-you ethos and for a general openness to spiritual experimentation. In addition to seeking combinations that would permit some contrasts and comparisons, these choices reflect the cities where I had academic, personal, or yoga colleagues or friends who could help me to see the cities as insiders see them. Before I received the grant that powered this project, I used its guiding questions to conduct a pilot project in Victoria, where I live.

Beyond the official project activities described above, three additional sources of data should be noted. First, as an adjunct to my roughly ten hours of studio practice per week since 2013, I have always tried to practise in any city where I have found myself for more than a few days during conferences or holidays. This face-to-face exposure was augmented by practising with nearly a dozen online instructors from various yoga denominations for about two years during pandemic-related studio closures. I have also participated in nine weekend conferences or workshop retreats in British Columbia led by authorized experts within the international Ashtanga scene. These events are common in yogaland and typically include a high-profile guest teacher who spends between two and seven days with between eight and thirty students. Workshops are often held in retreat centres or in a local studio. The guest teacher usually leads social events; group practice; a textual study of some kind, typically focused on parts of the *Bhagavad Gita* or the *Yoga Sutras*; and sessions devoted to some aspect of asana practice, such as backbends, or to some aspect of the broader yoga tradition, such as pranayama (breath work), chanting, or Sanskrit.

Second, I teach an undergraduate course on the people and politics of postural yoga at the University of Victoria in a city well known among North American sociologists for having the highest proportion (over 60 per cent) of people who tell pollsters that they have no religion – the so-called "religious nones." I have taught this course three times, and each time I have learned a great deal from my students about the kinds of yoga that many of them practise as members of a generation of which, in Victoria, roughly 75 per cent is made up of nones. I have also learned about the meanings of spirituality, religion, wellness, and Asia for a cohort of people who have mostly grown up with no specific religious affiliation, who are able to travel more than people in previous generations, and who are witnessing the world's climate spin out of control.

Whereas I grew up afraid of a sudden and devastating nuclear war between two recalcitrant superpowers, the world of my students and my twenty-two-year-old son is quite different. Does an embodied physical practice mean something particular for people who are healthier than they will probably ever be but who live on a planet that might be dying? What might participation in a practice that is storied as ancient and timeless mean for people who often feel rootless? These are questions addressed in the course, and the answers that students have provided over the years have helped to round out my understanding of postural yoga.

Third, early during our fieldwork, it became clear that the teacher training, or TT, experience was a ritualized threshold crossed not just by teachers but also by advanced students. The 200-hour TT programs offered all over the world and credentialed by the Yoga Alliance mark the beginning of many practitioners' serious engagement with yoga.

Since I kept hearing about these programs in interviews and focus groups but also through advertisements at nearly every studio, I decided to enrol in a four-month, 200-hour "traditional vinyasa" TT in Victoria (an "RYS-200" program approved by the Yoga Alliance). This training entailed many two- or three-day weekends spent in a studio from 7:00 a.m. until about 5:00 p.m. While there, I learned about yoga-related aspects of anatomy and physiology; key portions of the *Yoga Sutras*; the ethical quandaries that teachers face regarding their relationships with students; the history of postural yoga in India and the West; and the main chants associated with postural yoga in the Krishnamacharya tradition. In addition to videos and lectures, most TTs include a group-teaching assessment and both written and oral exams related to anatomy, Sanskrit posture names, and philosophical concepts.

The T T also introduced me to ways of adjusting students, of helping them to pair their breathing with their movement, and of responding to student interest in the more-than-physical elements of yoga. In my T T, students practised their adjustment and pedagogical techniques on one another and on friends and family, but we also spent several hours "shadowing" senior teachers as they taught classes in the Mysore style of Ashtanga vinyasa yoga. This component allowed T T participants to observe the ways that expert teachers adjusted students of all levels and to get advice from these teachers about our own adjustment styles.

Early in the writing process, I decided not to write only for the yoga scholars whose work in philology, history, sociology, or political science has shaped my own thinking. I respect them very much but opted not to use the specialized jargon, large numbers of parenthetical references, and dense prose that are the hallmarks of specialist writing.[18] Nonetheless, I also decided that I could not write a strictly "popular" book aimed at practitioners with no interest in debates about society, history, or politics.

Instead, I have opted to translate the issues of interest to scholars into language that I hope makes sense to all readers and simultaneously to translate the concerns of practitioners into language that is meaningful to those who study these subjects.

This is a tall order, to be sure. The first risk is that students and teachers may not like when their own feelings and perspectives regarding yoga, the sacred, the uniqueness of Asian spiritualities, and so on are rendered in the analytical language of scholarship. The second risk is that scholars might be disappointed that I do not rely on the vernacular unique to our fields, with terrifying boundary-making words such as "hermeneutical," "ontological," "discursive," "biopolitical," and "epistemological" used as though their meanings are self-evident (they rarely are, but we pretend otherwise). In a book about an extremely popular practice that is also the meeting place of complex social dynamics, I believe that my approach is worthwhile, although ultimately that is for readers to decide.

Speaking of Risks and Adults

There are hundreds, if not thousands, of classical and medieval philosophical and asana-related texts that have yet to be translated, much less interpreted, so the foundational work on the trajectories of yoga from ancient to modern South Asia and beyond will continue for decades.[19] Moreover, work on yoga in modern Western societies is by definition relatively recent, if expanding quickly. Again, readers interested in these lines of research can consult the endnotes. Suffice it to say that I admire these thinkers a great deal, and I hope that *Yogalands: In Search of Practice on the Mat and in the World* makes a small contribution to the conversation about modern yoga.

I have an interest in reflecting seriously on what it might mean for practitioners to move beyond what we might think of as an innocent approach to their practice. I sympathize with insiders for whom this departure from innocence is a hard sell since I appreciate the purpose or value of enchanting and all-encompassing religious and spiritual practices. In fact, initially, the title of this book was to be *Yoga for Adults*. I gave up this idea after I realized that it unfairly presupposed that other people would understand what I meant by adulthood. Nonetheless, this earlier title echoes a deep curiosity about the ways that insiders often have innocent (and sometimes well-fortified) views of religious or spiritual practices that become less and less tenable as we age and learn more about these practices and the cultures that produce them.

Critical inquiry into modern postural yoga – that is to say, the normal approach that scholars are supposed to take to all topics – can be threatening to practitioners. In 2010, Mark Singleton published *Yoga Body: The Origins of Modern Posture Practice*, in which he contended that modern yoga does not, as teachers often say or imply, continue an unbroken 5,000-year-old Indian tradition. Instead, he argued, it has roots not only in ancient esoteric and ascetic Indian religious and physical practices and texts but also in nineteenth- and twentieth-century European exercise traditions and resistance to British colonial control of India. Responses to his book from many practitioners were (and often still are) quite critical, underlining just how difficult it can be to challenge orthodoxy. I am a devoted practitioner but one who takes the argument that Singleton makes seriously. In general, it seems to me that whatever errors or exaggerations might exist in his massively influential book, subsequent research into postural yoga's development over the past several centuries has generally confirmed his basic argument. In any event, I am much less interested in offering a criticism or defence of Singleton's theory of the multiple roots of modern postural yoga than I am in documenting how practitioners respond to challenges to the core stories, practices, and leaders on which modern yoga – whether it takes place in an Ashtanga shala in Dallas or at a YMCA in Edmonton – depends.

Consider the following hypothetical scenarios (and I ask readers to forgive the fanciful conjectures):

The figure of Mahavatar Babaji, a supposedly ageless Himalayan yogi, looms large in the life story of Paramahansa Yogananda, who founded the Self-Realization Fellowship and wrote *Autobiography of a Yogi* (1946). Imagine that historians discover the diary of Lahiri Mahasaya (the guru of Sri Yukteswar Giri, who inspired Yogananda). *What if*, in this diary, Mahayasa outlines how he fabricated the story of his encounters with immortal Babaji of Indic legend? What might that mean for followers of Yogananda or practitioners of Kriya Yoga?

What if historians discover an exchange of letters between Krishnamacharya, European linguists, and officials of the Mysore Palace in the 1930s and this exchange shows that the founder of modern yoga covered up evidence that many asanas in use today were invented outside of South Asia or the Hindu orbit, originating instead with Europeans, Adivasis, Buddhists, Egyptians, or Chinese merchants?

Finally, *what if* several compelling scientific studies of the health claims often made about postural yoga conclude that it has only a placebo effect or, indeed, even an overall negative effect? What if this effect is so clear that the World Health Organization issues a stern warning about asana practice?

These far-fetched examples might be difficult to imagine, but it is nevertheless worthwhile for practitioner-readers to reflect on their initial reactions to these thought experiments.

Entering the world of postural yoga is experienced by so many, including myself, as a kind of conversion experience. When I tell colleagues about my experience of yoga, they recognize the predictable arc of a conversion story: "I once was lost but now am found; was blind, but now I see." There was the debilitated, wincing, limping me, then there was that long staircase, and now there is the relatively robust me writing this book. Try as I might to alter the tone or organization of the story, it continues to have a suffering and redemption structure indicative of the Christian hymn "Amazing Grace." When academic peers ask me about yoga, I usually caution them that they are about to hear this kind of story. I suppose that I offer this warning to diminish the awkward silences that might ensue as peers wonder whether I have forsaken my usual critical posture.

Among people who have experienced this dramatic before-and-after experience, there is often, and quite understandably, a strong resistance to subjecting their communities and practices to scrutiny, lest it spoil the spiritual transformations and physical healing that they have felt. Perhaps, they worry, disenchantment is the natural result of turning the scholarly spotlight on a yoga community or, for that matter, on a beloved family system, religious institution, sports team, nation, or art form. In response to the threat posed by dispassionate analysis, the temptation is to seal the experience, the teachers, the lore, and the tradition into a black box, never to be pried open by outsiders.

Scholars naturally lament this resistance since it makes it more difficult to describe, understand, or interpret certain experiences. But relegating these conversion experiences to black boxes may cost practitioners something too. After all, there is at least a chance that critical engagement with these profound experiences could enhance them. I for one am not interested in maintaining a practice if the convictions to which it might be connected wither under scrutiny. I suspect that practitioners who have come this far in the book will also be confident that their passion for postural yoga can withstand and perhaps be strengthened by outside inquiry.

It seems to me that a post-innocence yoga, or a yoga for adults, may permit a more profound pursuit of the deeper potential of practice; I suspect that the same thing would hold for a Christianity for adults, an America for adults, or a Smith family for adults. This is not to say that it is easy to abandon the initial enchantment that might have drawn students into a practice in the first place. But perhaps there are certain rewards only possible through transcending what we might think of as a child's yoga, or for that matter, as a child's Christianity, America, Smith family, and so forth.

Psychotherapist and senior Kripalu Yoga figure Stephen Cope writes that North American yoga students often hear and say, "Yoga is about getting out of your head and into your body."[20] I have heard versions of this maxim countless times since 2013, the most famous of which is Ashtanga guru Pattabhi Jois's oft-repeated contention that Ashtanga yoga is 99 per cent practice and 1 per cent theory. Cope argues that this focus on the physical body over what happens in the mind or spirit has also resulted in a certain anti-intellectualism in modern postural yoga communities. There is a "relentless bias in American yoga against the systematic study and understanding of yoga metaphysics ... [which] has created an enormous amount of confusion about what the practice of yoga really is."[21]

I see my role not as adjudicating what yoga really is but as reflecting on what it also is. Still, Cope's argument about the anti-intellectual bias in yogaland seems fair. However, this common self-imposed limitation is not surprising. It grows out of the fact that yoga in North America is a stew with many ingredients: dualism and monism, North American spiritualism and New Thought, theosophy, materialism, Buddhism, Hinduism, quantum physics, a sizable helping of neo-Tantrism, and a "self-spirituality"[22] that has emerged as conventional religions have declined. So those interested in teasing apart the many forces shaping the studios that they might frequent or the online "yogalebrities" whom they might follow face a great challenge.[23]

Cope notes that the antipathy in yogaland with regard to serious scholarship on the practices that many yogis love reflects a misreading of the history of yoga, a tradition in which advanced intellectual engagement has always been highly valued: "Yogis ... do not consider being intellectual different from being physical: in classical yoga, anything that belongs to the realm of the phenomenal world – which the mind manifestly does – is seen as a physical activity."[24]

I am aware that some readers will not be practitioners and that some may be deeply suspicious of postural yoga. That is as it should be. I hope that these readers will nonetheless gain something from thinking about this massively popular North American practice. Just as inquiry need not destroy beloved practices, it also need not connote or lead to commitment.

As well, a great many practitioners simply enjoy the physical healing or pleasure that yoga can deliver and feel no need at all to scratch its surface or to wonder how it is related to the societies in which it is embedded. They may not share my sense of adulthood not just as a stage of life that one enters around one's twentieth year but also as a state of mind in which one becomes acutely aware of – and then, perhaps, tries to balance – contradictory feelings, experiences, and responsibilities. For the record, however, I have in mind these kinds of contradictions:

- The United States is a beacon of liberty, creativity, and opportunity, yet it is a deeply divided society on the verge of collapse due to racism, nationalism, and populism.
- Canada is the home of peace, order, and good governance, yet it is a smug, fragmented settler colonial state that is suicidally dependent on natural resource extraction.
- Christianity is the religion of a radical Jewish pacifist and prophet committed to spiritual and political liberation, yet it is inextricably entangled in some of the worst forms of colonialism, misogyny, and violence ever seen in human history.

I do not have a preferred sense of what a yoga for adults might look like for other people. However, from years of talking with practitioners and non-practitioners alike, I can tell that even before picking up this book, people could probably complete at least one half or perhaps both halves of a "Yoga is this, yet it is also that" binary. Regardless of what brings a reader to these pages, I hope that a serious but also playful inquiry into yoga in North America will help to make conversations about yoga both a little less innocent and a little more open-ended than they often are. But beyond this aim, it seems to me that it is valuable to cultivate an ability to recognize that we embrace numerous ideas in our minds and that we engage in many practices with our bodies that are incongruous if not mutually exclusive. The point is not to correct this state of affairs so much as it is to understand it.

I confess that I usually end my undergraduate course on yoga with a sutra of my own: curiosity is the most important asana. I imagine that it makes some of my twenty-year-old students roll their eyes, but I think that it is true.

INTRODUCTION

It seems to me that the best way to address what it might mean to think about and through postural yoga is to be curious about the problems often associated with yoga in contemporary North America. By considering some of the major fault lines running through modern postural yoga, we can see the complexity within issues that might seem simple on the surface. In chapter 1, I reflect on the common claim that yoga is apolitical. Depending on who is making this argument, it is meant either as an indictment or as a selling point. But in what ways is yoga political or apolitical, and how does this issue matter? It turns out that one's response to this dilemma tells us a lot about what one thinks about both the core mandate of yoga and the greatest problems that vex our societies.

In chapter 2, I address the thorny claim that yoga is spiritual but not religious. I am not interested in arguing that it is actually spiritual, religious, both, or neither. Rather, an exploration of this often heard but rarely examined claim tells us how it came to pass that spirituality (and the individual) came to eclipse religion (and institutions) as the key metaphor to use when thinking about supernatural experience and human transformation.

In chapter 3, we move out of the mind and into the body since it was really the wounded body that took centre stage in so many conversations during fieldwork, just as it has during my years of practice and study. I was touched by the vulnerability that people shared with me; it demonstrated the many ways that "the body keeps the score," to use Bessel van der Kolk's evocative phrase.[25] We also heard innumerable stories about how postural yoga practices had transformed these soft, wounded bodies – these fragile objects – into vehicles for healing. The body clearly also settles the score. This restored yoga body becomes, then, the access point par excellence for the higher spiritual or religious promises of yoga.

In chapter 4, I introduce superheroes. The yoga of Patanjali, author of the *Yoga Sutras*, is dualistic in the sense that there are distinct forces at work in the universe, namely purusha (consciousness) and prakriti (material nature). The emphasis for Patanjali is on withdrawing from ordinary life to manage one's mind and body through a variety of yogic disciplines. Practice assiduously, reduce attachments, come to know the correct relationship between purusha and prakriti and between one's atman (higher self) and Brahman (ultimate reality). So far, so good, or at least this is the general story that is told at most studios when yoga philosophy is introduced. These are objectives that I consider later in this book.

What is almost never discussed explicitly – and in interviews it was clear that this topic was not of much interest – is the fact that the *Yoga Sutras* includes perhaps twenty times as many sutras about special powers as about asanas. It is odd that these dramatic powers (including invisibility, shape-shifting, and mind reading) are almost never mentioned in yogaland, given their clear importance in this brief "bible of yoga." However, it is also the case that even if teachers and students do not speak openly about the special powers attributed to gifted yogis in the *Yoga Sutras*, yogaland is arguably full of siddhas (perfected beings) and jivanmuktas (superpeople). These beautiful creatures can be found in magazines and at the front of many classes, but they are also next to you in class, silently displaying their gifts through effortless asana or pranayama.

In chapter 5, we travel to India, or at least to the idea of India as it circulates within yogaland. We take a circuitous route through two controversies that may threaten the aura of the subcontinent. The scandals that emerged shortly before and during the #MeToo movement certainly forced not just practitioners but indeed entire lineages to reconsider the ways that they imagine India, Asia, and the authority of teachers. What freight do we ask these places to carry, and to what end? For many of the people we met, India is first and foremost a symbol – but of what, and why is it needed? Is India's romanticized image sustainable now that no one can claim not to know that widespread sexual misconduct was made possible by gurus who used their ascribed power to violate vulnerable people (mostly women)?

In recent years, it has become somewhat more difficult for affluent, white Westerners to pick and choose those elements of subaltern cultures that suit their personal or commercial interests. The truth and reconciliation process in Canada and the Black Lives Matter movement in the United States have – to use a phrase that seems anachronistic – raised the consciousness of many people in our societies. This is not to say that either society has banished racism but rather that its ugliest expressions are increasingly pushed to the margins (especially in Canada, it seems). As a result of these shifts in Canadian and American life, non-Indians might be inclined to think more seriously about whether it is appropriate to selectively take on Indic ideas, language, and symbolism in their personal or spiritual lives.

It is unusual to think of the #MeToo and cultural appropriation controversies together, but in my view they weaken what I call a load-bearing wall of modern postural yoga, namely its link to ancient India. I was struck by the fact that for many yogis – perhaps even most – these crises seem well compartmentalized and do not threaten their practice. But why not?

Throughout this book, I reflect on the idea that yoga studios offer practitioners an alternative to a regular world that is excessively loud, fast, and dirty – to introduce a refrain that I use throughout the book and that is gleaned from interviews as well as from the common aesthetic of so many studios. The yoga mat is promoted as an oasis of calm, a place of retreat, where people can temporarily leave the world behind. Sometimes the anti-world features of yogaland are critiques of the world, and sometimes they are escapes from that world. In any event, understanding the relationship between world and anti-world is crucial not just for understanding postural yoga but also for understanding the many objectionable features of our world that so many North Americans manage through yoga. The ways that we see, critique, and sometimes escape this world reveal a great deal about my main interests: yoga, our society, and ourselves.

CHAPTER ONE

The Mat Is Not Always the Territory

At the beginning of many postural yoga classes, teachers often ask students to stand at the front of their mats, with eyes shut and hands at heart centre, so that everyone in the class can synchronize their breath, chant "om," and recite an invocation in Sanskrit. Students are often encouraged to "breathe in peace, exhale, release." Teachers might explain these ritualized actions as ways to "centre yourselves, take a break from your regular lives, be at peace with your body, set an intention, give yourselves the privilege of attending to your own needs for the next hour," and so forth.

The scenes described above will be familiar to anyone who has entered the utopian alternative space that I think of, following Patrick McCartney, as yogaland.[1] Whether I am practising in Barcelona, Sydney, Victoria, New York, Göttingen, Waterloo, or Winnipeg, I know that the owners, managers, and teachers have gone to great lengths to make sure that I am extracted from my regular life and ushered into a new world. The studio is an anti-world in the sense that it subverts an outside world that is often experienced as too loud, fast, and dirty. These anti-worlds create what anthropologist Sarah Strauss calls "oasis regimes," or alternatives to one's normal life.[2] Of course, elements of the outside world continue to influence these quiet, slow, clean spaces, but for now it is important to note that these spaces are designed to allow practitioners to escape.[3]

One way to understand a common set of practices that can entail breathing and speaking in unison, standing in a clean and orderly space, and holding one's hands in a prayer position is to think about what problem this set of practices is trying to address.

The consensus among the teachers and students I met is that these practices are aimed first and foremost at alleviating suffering. On the surface, students are drawn to the promise that yoga might help to heal a bad back, depression, cancer, or arthritis. Below the surface, there might be a wish to address the more complex emotional or traumatic wounds that are manifested, finally, in one's body.

Some ambitious teachers – many of whom readers will meet throughout this book – also introduce students to yogic accounts of the ultimate origin of our suffering, which is often framed as avidya (ignorance of reality).[4] For our purposes, it is worthwhile to note that it is quite understandable that many practitioners – and even graduates of teacher-training programs – may conclude that yoga is fundamentally apolitical. Indeed, Patanjali's yoga could be seen as a handmaiden of the status quo precisely because of its focus on the self's realization of truth rather than on the promotion of some clear idea of social justice. At least to many outside observers, postural yoga lacks the world-fixing ambitions associated with Christian liberation theology, not to mention with some forms of hip-hop and rock and roll. All of these practices have been commercialized or leashed, of course, but they have not entirely lost the edge that they had at their inceptions. It is unclear whether postural yoga ever had or might yet develop this activist orientation.

Of course, the other reason that people might assume yoga to be apolitical is that it seems to be entirely at home in an individualistic, neoliberal, consumer society. Indeed, the recent growth of postural yoga in the West owes a great deal to its prominence within celebrity culture and to its promotion by "athleisure" brands such as Lululemon and Alo. How could those who embrace a practice so neatly aligned with the interests of a rapacious capitalism be interested in altering the political world?

In this chapter, I want to suggest that postural yoga is and arguably has always been inherently political. In fact, the most common political feature

29

of postural yoga is its promise to offer an escape from a loud, fast, and dirty world. Even though many practitioners evade political questions on the mat and in studios, politics follow them there.

The Body Politic: From Gross to Subtle

To explain what I mean when I suggest that yoga is inherently political, I will use a contrast – often invoked in yogaland – between the gross (physical or lower) and the subtle (spiritual or higher) bodies. These are just two aspects of our personhoods, and yogic practices often promise to help us cultivate the correct relationship between them.[5] I frame these metaphors somewhat differently, using them as a means to draw our attention to what we might call the gross as opposed to subtle levels of the body politic. As in the human self, the relationship between these two aspects of one's body takes the form not of a stark binary but of a spectrum.

When I suggest that yoga is political in the gross sense, I am referring to the common use of the word. Consider a few of the most obvious moments when yoga has entered the gross political realm. Each of these examples reflects different aspects both of the societies in which the controversies arose and of the forms of yoga that took centre stage. This is not the place to tease out the many implications of these incidents, but the endnotes do offer readers a sense of where else to look. My real interest in this brief section is to provide a snapshot of the many ways that yoga has been a key concern for politicians around the world for decades.

The best examples of this concern come from contemporary India, where Prime Minister Narendra Modi and supporters such as billionaire yogi Baba Ramdev work to remind Indians that postural yoga is India's gift to humanity. Indeed, in India there is an official government body, the Ministry of Ayurveda, Yoga and Naturopathy, Unani, Siddha and Homoeopathy (AYUSH), devoted to the regulation and promotion of five Indian healing modalities: Ayurveda, Yoga, Unani, Siddha, and Homeopathy.[6] On the ministry's website, one finds practical advice for how to avoid and treat COVID-19 through Ayurvedic medicine, for example.

As the burgeoning popularity of postural yoga around the world became clear, the Indian government increasingly integrated postural yoga into its broader branding endeavours. In addition to the work of the Ministry of AYUSH, these efforts are most apparent in the government's creation, promotion, and publication in 2015 of the *Common Yoga Protocol* and in its establishment in 2014 of the International Day of Yoga, first observed in 2015. Through these two initiatives, Modi and his Bharatiya Janata Party celebrate yoga's inalienable Indian origins and essence. In print, online, and in video, the protocol has been widely circulated in India and across social media.

Through the protocol, students are taught not just a sequence of postures but also the spiritual, intellectual, and physiological value of asana practice. For example, in the *Common Yoga Protocol*, we read,

> The science of Yoga has its origin thousands of years ago, long before the first religion or belief systems were born …
>
> Yoga is widely considered as an "immortal cultural outcome" of the Indus Saraswati Valley Civilisation – dating back to 2700 BC – and has proven itself to cater to both material and spiritual uplift of humanity. A number of seals and fossil remains of Indus Saraswati Valley Civilisation with Yogic motifs and figures performing *Yoga s dhana* suggest the presence of Yoga in ancient India. The seals and idols of mother Goddess are suggestive of *Tantra* Yoga. The presence of Yoga is also available in folk traditions, Vedic and Upanishadic heritage, Buddhist and Jain traditions, *Darshanas*, epics of Mahabharata including Bhagawadgita and Ramayana, theistic traditions of Shaivas, Vaishnavas and Tantric traditions. Though Yoga was being practiced in the pre-Vedic period, the great sage Maharishi Patanjali systematised and codified the then existing Yogic practices, its meaning and its related knowledge through Patanjali's *Yoga Sutras* …
>
> Yoga is essentially a path to liberation from all bondage. However, medical research in recent years has uncovered many physical and mental benefits that Yoga offers, corroborating the experiences of millions of practitioners …
>
> Yogic Practice shall start with a prayer or prayerful mood to enhance the benefits of practice.[7]

I suspect that it is difficult for many readers in Western liberal democracies to imagine our governments becoming equally involved in efforts to promote analogous religious or spiritual traditions or practices. Modi launched the International Day of Yoga at the United Nations in 2014 with an impassioned political speech that spelled out the value of yoga as a spiritual and physical intervention.[8] The word "political," of course, usually has negative connotations, but I use it here to mean organized efforts to govern a country. Part of this undertaking involves the promotion of a galvanizing story – we could use the word "ideology" instead – about the way that a particular group of people came into being, what challenges they face, and how they ought to behave among themselves and toward others. Yoga has been integrated at a formal level into the broader story that the Indian state tells its citizens, as well as the world, about what it means to be Indian and what the society has given the world. I mention these efforts here not to dispute the claims made in the *Common Yoga Protocol* but to draw attention to ways that the document presents to the world an image of India in which specific religious and spiritual ideas and practices are central to Indian society's identity.

Critics have observed that since 1947, the post-independence dream of India has always been haunted by the fact that one community vastly outnumbers the others. These critics allege that Modi and his ministers use the global interest in yoga to offer the Indian public a unifying symbol but one that nonetheless marginalizes India's roughly 200 million Muslims (approximately 15 per cent of the Indian population).[9] Some Muslims resent the way yoga's framing as an indispensable element of Indian Identity alienates those Muslims who feel that postures such as urdhva hastasana (raised hands pose; see figure 1.1), which is the beginning of surya namaskara (sun salutation pose), both smack of idolatry in the form of sun worship and convey the message that Muslims who may not follow yogic spirituality do not really belong in (or to) India.[10]

Although Indian politicians employ religious leaders, ideas, imagery, and events to bolster their political careers in explicit ways that very few US or Canadian politicians would consider, yoga has been involved in North American politics too. In fact, I first became interested in applying my professional training to my relatively new personal interest in postural yoga in 2015 when Christy Clark, then premier of British Columbia, opted to celebrate the International Day of Yoga by holding a massive asana class on a Vancouver bridge early on a Sunday morning. She had every reason to think

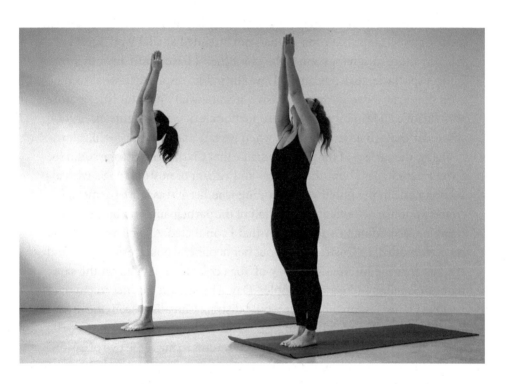

Figure 1.1
Urdhva hastasana (raised hands pose)

that such an event would allow her to capitalize on the tremendous popularity of yoga in Vancouver, on the region's burgeoning Indo-Canadian community, and on India's expanding economic ambitions.

She seemed genuinely stupefied and actually rather wounded by the fact that immediately after she had made her announcement, the public reaction was loud and almost uniformly negative. I had never admired her party's policies or principles and would not have participated in the event myself (since it would feel unnatural to me to practise in public). I might have been a curious spectator; but even if I had not attended at all, I would not have had any more misgivings about the event than I have about any other big-budget spectacle, such as Canada Day. The public response to what seemed – on the surface – to be an inoffensive, if somewhat opportunistic, gesture was vitriolic and (in my view) disproportionate. It was, nonetheless, a good reminder that what we talk about when we talk about yoga is, well, a lot.

Below the surface of the public ridicule that Clark received, one could see strong stereotypes about the silliness and elitism of postural yoga, with almost no one in the public debate asking whether it was fair to demean extremely popular activities to which half of the participants attribute spiritual meaning, according to a 2017 survey that I conducted. As well, the backlash reflected both deep frustrations about her neoliberal policy orientation and the fact that the International Day of Yoga coincidentally fell on the same date as Canada's Indigenous Peoples' Day. The latter led critics to contend that the asana class on the bridge would distract Canadians from the urgent need for reconciliation with Indigenous communities. What led me to write about this controversy was the fact that the events to mark the two occasions were 8 kilometres and several hours apart, with the asana class being only one of many major public events in the city that weekend. In other words, people could easily have attended both events if they had wanted. Under the weight of the unanticipated backlash, Clark cancelled the event within a week of launching it.[11]

In Encinitas, California, postural yoga also became the subject of public, political, and legal attention. In this case – emerging in 2013 and resolved finally in 2015 – an evangelical Christian parent objected to the fact that her daughter was involved in a yoga class in her school.[12] The class was part of a program funded by the Jois Foundation, associated with the founder of the Ashtanga yoga lineage. The case made news across the country, with most stories revolving around whether yoga postures could be taught to elementary school children in a manner that did not run afoul of the US constitutional provisions prohibiting the promotion of religion in public educational institutions. In the end, the program continued, but the teachers had to assure the school and the parents that the students were not asked to pray, were not introduced to the philosophy or history of Indic yoga traditions, and were not taught the Sanskrit terms for the postures; for example, instead of padmasana (full lotus pose; see figure 1.2), children were taught "criss-cross applesauce."

The use of postural yoga within the US prison system offers another example of yoga's presence in the gross political arena. It might surprise some readers to learn that yoga programs are quite common in prisons, not just in the United States but elsewhere as well.[13] Many argue that the US prison industrial complex – an appropriate metaphor, given the burgeoning privatization of correctional facilities there – is a powerfully conservative force in a society characterized by racism, white supremacy, classism, and sexual violence.[14] Although there might be an intrinsic value to yoga programs for inmates, critics such as Andrea Jain and Farah Godrej share a concern about the ways that postural yoga may stifle the dissent that would otherwise reveal a deeply dysfunctional society.[15]

Moving toward the more subtle end of the spectrum, we can look to the work of Andrea Jain, who is well known for her books *Selling Yoga* and *Peace Love Yoga*. Jain is aware that yoga students and teachers regularly speak of their practices in terms of personal transformation and wellness.

When I ask students and teachers about the connection between the broader world and what they do in their studios, they are likely to give me the same look that one might see if one were to ask an ardent home gardener how their garden influences climate change. The gardener might observe that their lush oasis must have a net positive impact on climate change variables (and no doubt it does), although this impact was not really what led them to the garden centre in the first place. Similarly, yoga practitioners may

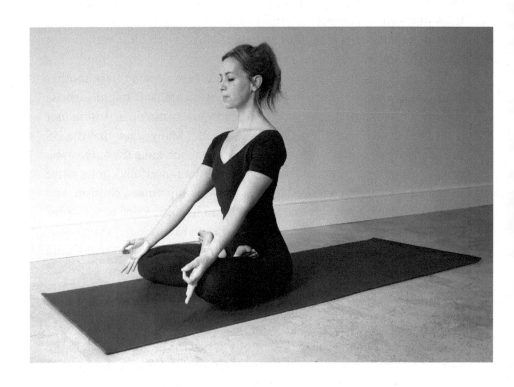

Figure 1.2
Padmasana (full lotus pose)

say that the world in general is improved when yoga students are healthier, happier, calmer, and more reflective, but as Jain observes, the social or political impacts are, as it were, downstream benefits that are not clearly identified and that are difficult to demonstrate after the fact.

However, not all practitioners are satisfied with the vague pursuit of "good vibes" and "positive energy." They want to address political issues directly. When I asked teachers and students about organized efforts to connect postural yoga and social justice endeavours, several examples were offered: the Yoga Gives Back charity raises funds to support women and children in India; the New Leaf Foundation teaches yoga and meditation techniques to marginalized youth in the Greater Toronto Area; Off the Mat supports grassroots change around the world; the Yoga Alliance offers advice and resources to help make postural yoga more accessible to a wider range of students; and many yoga studios raise funds for "diversity scholarships" through lower-cost community classes, the proceeds from which support the regular membership fees of marginalized students.[16]

As one leading figure within Toronto's Modo (hot yoga) community remarked,

Modo has something called Karma classes, and all the Modo studios have to have them. And all the money that you raise, you have to donate all the money. Like you can't take any to pay a teacher or anything. And I think across the Modo community and the twenty years or whatever we've raised close to $10 million for charity. So we work closely with the David Suzuki Foundation [for environmental causes].

But more recently, we've given a lot of money to Black Lives Matter groups and all, all different communities. So part of the Modo, I don't know if it's like [Modo's] philosophy or whatever, it has a huge give-back component. And the studios are all Bullfrog power [a green energy system within Ontario], voc- [volatile organic compound-] free paint, [and] we clean with all natural cleaning materials. These are really important principles for us.

Commenting on the contributions to the broader world that are made by the Isha yoga community, which is associated with the Indian yogi Sadhguru, a US community member observed,

37

There's a huge social outreach component within the work of the [Isha] Foundation. So we have three main social outreach initiatives for health, environment, and education. And this is something that [Sadhguru] said, "Asking a hungry man to meditate is obscene because a hungry man is thinking about his next meal. He's not thinking about meditation." So this is where, you know, a big component of our work is to bring people the basic survival needs before we move them into meditation.

There are many other examples of noteworthy social justice projects associated with postural yoga communities in North America.

Like me, Jain is alive to and appreciates their work, but she raises questions about the centrality of these movements within the larger yoga ecosystem, so to speak. Such activities do occur, as any consideration of bulletin boards and email and Facebook campaigns common in yogaland will prove. However, Jain asks about both the prominence and impact of these activities and about just how explicitly or effectively these events link what happens in a studio space with broader social problems, which are mostly produced by capitalism, in her view. She contends – and I agree, based on my findings – that the primary objective in most studios is personal improvement, not social change. Consequently, postural yoga may not have an appreciable impact on the negative features of modern life, such as violence, unemployment, homelessness, hopelessness, environmental destruction, and the suicide and opioid epidemics.

Capitalism might generate much of the suffering that leads people to a yoga studio, but it also supplies an explanation for studios' emphasis on individual wellness over societal wellness. Since the studios need to generate an income to pay their rent, teacher fees, and insurance, devoting a lot of time to social justice campaigns would reduce the time and energy available for student recruitment, new class offerings, and lucrative teacher-training programs. With a few exceptions, these communities are structured as businesses, after all, and understandably have to survive in a commercial environment.

In addition, when new students talk about what brought them into a studio, they almost never list resisting authoritarianism, increasing access to abortion services, or reducing income inequality, even if they might feel strongly about these issues as personal or social priorities. As I discuss throughout the book, their main motivation is health and recovery from traumas and the damages inflicted by a loud, fast, and dirty world. As businesses, studios respond to the immediate needs of their clients and to the administrative and financial contingencies of their organization (e.g., the cost of rent and insurance).

Although the studio owners and teachers I met were not actively hostile to a greater emphasis on social or political justice issues, most students neither expect nor demand these features. The lack of such explicit undertakings in yoga communities does raise the concerns of critics. As Farah Godrej claims, an involvement in postural yoga may lead a practitioner to become "amenable to arrogations of power, absorbed in pursuing her free choice of yoga practice, disinterested in questioning the broader structures that produce differential outcomes." In other words, yoga may relax and distract people so much that they cease to notice or to care much about our societies' many flaws. As a result, to use Jain's useful term, any subversion of the status quo may be merely a "gesture" as opposed to a pragmatic solution with lasting impact.[17]

Does a yoga practice with no explicit intention to alter the world outside of the studio function in the ways that Karl Marx argued that religion functions? Do both yoga and religion function as an "opium of the people"? It is useful to remember that his perspective on religion is often misunderstood. Here is the phrase in context: "Religion is the sigh of the oppressed creature, the heart of a heartless world and the soul of soulless conditions. It is the opium of the people."[18] Religion provides relief from the crushing, soul-destroying material conditions in which people live. It represents their attempts to remain human ("the heart of a heartless world") – which Marx appreciated. It can also be a distracting illusion that naturalizes the injustices of this world and that discourages solidarity and justice seeking – effects that he did not appreciate. His account of religion is more compassionate, more subtle, than many people imagine; it is possible that he might have adopted the same perspective on yoga if he had encountered its contemporary Western variants.

When I raised Jain's (and Marx's) critique with Canadian yoga scholar and teacher Braj, his response braided together Marxist and yogic threads:

I've had ... racialized students get very upset when I [argue that yoga might distract people from an unfair political reality]. Just recently, I had a yoga teacher tell me: "This is the time I need where there's no politics, there's no moral questions, I'm just taking care of myself." I'm like, "You should be doing that all the time." But then you'd have to deal with these moral and political questions about injustice, and you'd have to get to the yamas [the restraints, the first limb of Patanjali's yoga]. You'd have to do all that kind of more radical work. But [the student in question] had internalized this [apolitical approach] to the point where she was like, "You know, I'm just going to do it in this space." So it's alarming to her to have to be political. Meanwhile, that's the only way that she is going to be the agent of her own, her own liberation. And we see this all the time. So then yoga becomes vacation.

I have seen this in my own life. Monday through Friday, I begin Mysore practice around 6:00 a.m. and spend roughly ninety minutes on the mat. It is common for Ashtanga yoga practitioners not to consume anything apart from coffee or tea before practice. So when I come home around 8:00 a.m., I am hungry and eager to have a shower. As well, as a generally anxious person, I am acutely aware that I have a long list of home and work tasks to tackle that day. Ordinarily, this combination of facts would constitute a recipe for extreme irritability, but in fact I return home with a deep sense of serenity. I must be quite irksome for my family in the morning.

Sometimes I will cross paths with my partner as she prepares for a full day at her extremely stressful job. When I arrive, a sizable portion of her mind is already in her office with her often seriously ill patients. As we pass one another, sometimes at the front door, it seems as though my world and her world are rotating at different speeds. I follow her, with my eyes or my feet, but I cannot keep up, so I often end up saying goodbye to her back as she lurches out the door to repair the world.

This lingering euphoria after practice is a unique kind of sweetness, and from the vantage point of the oasis that my practice offers me, so many other issues in our world seem less distressing. Certainly, after time at the shala, I am stronger, more flexible, and more relaxed, but two hours later, I join the same maelstrom that my partner entered earlier.[19] Perhaps predictably, I am inclined to argue that the problems that led me to seek the respite of my early morning anti-world become less oppressive to me through my practice. Of course, it is also possible that the true source of my personal and our global problems is rendered opaque – and thus much more formidable and perhaps even permanent – by my morning equanimity. Of these two, which is the most compelling account of the impact of yoga on the broader society of which I am a part? If I want to encourage a yoga for adults, I need to acknowledge that the jury is still out.

To demonstrate the final and perhaps most subtle way in which postural yoga in North America is inherently political, let us consider where people think they live.

Tara is a practitioner in Toronto. One could say that she lives under the aegis of forces such as patriarchy and capitalism, as all Canadian women do. Perhaps sometimes she feels oppressed by these forces, and sometimes she feels that she can master or tolerate them. As well, she is burdened in particular by some of the normal physical challenges that yoga teachers often hear about from their students.

These macro (global) and micro (physical) factors help us to imagine her on her mat, but it is also important to note that Tara lives in a city, a province, and a society (a) where people are just beginning to take seriously what it might mean to reconcile with Indigenous peoples, (b) where it is fairly difficult for her to get a handgun, (c) where her health care is ostensibly free, (d) where her society's democratic institutions are intact, (e) where her reproductive rights are affirmed, and (f) where virtually all of her friends and family live in a thin band of land from Vancouver Island to Newfoundland, as opposed to being distributed evenly across the continent.[20] We might think of these as the meso (societal) factors of her life.

There are, of course, many characteristics that meet on her mat, such as age, sexual orientation, gender identity, income level, education, and physical abilities, but the point is just that when she is deep in her practice, she is not only a depressed diabetic who is irritated by the patriarchy. She is also – quite importantly – a Canadian.

Having now met a great many Taras, I can report that most of them do not speak in general terms of yoga in Canada, yoga in the West, Iyengar yoga in the United States, or hot yoga in Los Angeles. Instead, the most important frames of reference are their own bodies or their own studios. For the people I met, one might say that whether the minds and bodies in question happen to be in Köln, Kelowna, Kendal, or Killeen is unimportant.

As I have observed in this chapter, there is a tendency in yogaland to frame yoga as being disconnected from or unconcerned with politics. Just as pervasive is the tendency to forget that yoga is practised in particular *places*. Yet we often forget about the distinctive national and even regional features of our fundamental assumptions about health, race, economics, and democracy.

By way of an illustration of this tendency to forget, I will share two stories that convey not only the importance of national, or what I call meso-level, factors but also the somewhat embarrassing personal innocence I brought with me into the field.

Steve and Donna Say the Unsayable at 35,000 Feet

On an Alaska Airlines flight from Seattle to Indianapolis, I found myself in the window seat, next to Steve and Donna, two retired teachers in their late sixties.

After some small talk, they asked about my project. Although I was taking a small risk by introducing religion and yoga into a conversation with strangers, it struck me as a good opportunity to practise communicating the basic issues that I would be thinking and writing about for the next year or two.

This part of the discussion went well. When I mentioned that the continued support for former US president Donald Trump among millions of Americans was one of the things that fascinated me, they both groaned slightly and shook their heads. Donna said in an exasperated tone, "Ohh, I *know*. He's awful. For the record, we can't stand him."

We talked for a while about some of my concerns regarding my government's approach to natural resource extraction as well as Indigenous reconciliation. At this point, it was a very conventional conversation based on a consensus about their former president, our shared frustrations with ineffectual politicians, and a world in trouble. I began to wonder which movie I would watch for the rest of the flight.

Then Steve said, "And this is hard because we're Republicans." Looking back on my fieldnotes, I am a little embarrassed that this comment confused me. In my defence, it was the very first day of our fieldwork, and I know almost no US Republicans and almost no Canadians with Republican sympathies. As the project expanded, I came to understand the specifically Canadian features of my imagination. At the same time as limiting my vision, these features alerted me to things that American colleagues might not have noticed.

"Sorry. Hang on. Do you mean you used to be Republicans? From what you just said, it sounded like you're really upset by what's happened to your party."

They sighed again. "No, you heard right. We totally disagree with him, and think he's a terrible person, but especially where we live, there is really no alternative. So, yes, we voted for him," Donna said. I was still processing this disclosure when she added, "I mean, among our friends and church people and just in our part of Indiana in general, it's basically impossible to support anyone else. Like, if we had a sign on our lawn for the Democrats? I mean, my God, I can't even imagine what might happen."

They noted that their daughters and sons-in-law are also Trump supporters. I asked what it was about him that appealed to them, and Steve said, "Well, it's mainly that they like what he did for their investment portfolio."

The conversation shifted. I told them that many of my Canadian peers are fascinated by the gun control debate. Since Indiana is an "open carry" state, meaning that one does not need a permit to carry a firearm in public, I thought that they would have an interesting perspective. They noted that their daughters and sons-in-law sometimes carry handguns. I could not restrain my curiosity, so I asked whether they lived in dangerous neighbourhoods or whether their jobs required it. Steve said, "No, they live in nice small towns."

Steve could see that I was confused. He seemed to notice what I think of as my Canada face, a perplexed and not entirely innocent befuddlement that often emerges when Canadians and Americans talk about their societies. I have heard that Americans find this face irritating, but Steve was not put off. He clarified, "Well, one of our daughters sometimes works with the fire department, though."

"Okay, so would she need a handgun for that?" I asked. "Maybe," Steve said. Donna cocked her head, squinted at him and said, "Well no, not really. Come on, Steve. Geez." She looked at me and confessed, "Honestly, no."

"Well," Steve added by way of a defence, "she likes to have a gun with her because sometimes she might find herself in sort of sketchy places."

There was an awkward pause in the conversation, and I thought I would take advantage of my actual (and tactical) Canadian naivete. "Can I float an idea past you? It's the kind of question you might expect from a foreign liberal, and so forgive me if it seems clueless. I promise we can go back to talking about yoga after."

"Sure," they said.

"Given what you've said about your daughters and sons-in-law and their handguns, I wonder if, when you say *sketchy*, you really mean *Black*?"

They both stiffened noticeably. After a pregnant pause, Donna looked at Steve, who breathed in and said, "Yes. I guess that is what I mean. I hate to say it, but yes, I guess that is the truth."

I played dumb again. Out of my Canada face came the question, "So, you're worried that in her fire department work, or just in life in general, she might come across a dangerous Black person in a sketchy area, or this person might come into her own nonsketchy and mostly white town? That's what worries her, and you?"

They both winced. "Ohhhh. Oh God," Donna said, as though Steve had just revealed their kinky sexual predilections.

Presumably to soften the story, Steve added, "Yes, I guess that's right. Just being honest. But it's not just Blacks. Also leftists and Antifa."

"Leftists and Antifa! Well! I don't think you have to worry about us. I mean, we might hit you with a rolled-up pamphlet, but otherwise, you're pretty safe."

This joke broke the tension that had been building over the previous half hour.

The horrified look on Donna's face had suggested that Steve had almost accidentally revealed something private, perhaps because it is hard to resist mid-flight intimacies with people whom you would never meet again and who had a sincere interest in your views.

As a relatively fair-skinned person of half Indo-Trinidadian origin, I generally pass for white, and throughout my life, the Canadian versions of Donna and Steve have taken me into their confidence and said things that they certainly would not have said if they had been aware of my personal history. On many occasions, these self-disclosures have created embarrassing experiences for me and my conversational partners when they have suddenly realized that it was a very bad idea to share their misgivings about mixed marriage, multiculturalism, or Indigenous reconciliation. I confess, regretfully, that I have often been quite contemptuous of such people.

Perhaps the fact that I was 35,000 feet above the earth and therefore unable to deliver a withering comeback to Steve's revelation led me to opt for a joke. Or perhaps this less aggressive response reflected the warmth of our conversation and my sense that we are all products of micro, meso, and macro influences that are expressed in ways that we often do not fully understand until someone asks us questions that social norms usually forbid.

Curtis Travels 5,000 Miles

Curtis, a thirty-five-year-old massage therapist and yoga teacher, noted that he had lived in Indianapolis for only a few years but had grown up in, worked in, and loved Hawaii for most of his life. When I asked what had brought him nearly 5,000 miles away from his home, he noted that as a private contractor in Hawaii, he had to pay for his own very bare-bones health insurance. So when his partner was offered a job in Indianapolis with robust coverage for both of them, they moved. There was nothing about Indy – relatives, friends, weather, exciting work opportunities for him – that made the move especially appealing, and he did not have a specific health concern that made him worry about his future. Quite the contrary was the case. This young, handsome, and preternaturally healthy man could easily be a model or a Lululemon brand ambassador.

In Hawaii, however, he worried about his health coverage regularly. "Because when you have to pay for your insurance out of pocket, [well,] I could see it was going up ... like 20 per cent every year." When I asked about his peers in the wellness industry, many of whom needed to purchase their own health coverage, he said, "I mean, [when they get sick,] they go to the hospital, but then somehow there's GoFundMe [a crowd-sourced online fundraising platform] ... They would raise, you know, enough money [to cover the treatment], but I was never someone who felt okay not having insurance because it can just totally destroy you financially."

A few moments earlier, when he told the story of moving from Hawaii to Indy for better health care coverage, I looked around the room and saw that everyone else present – all Americans – were nodding indifferently in recognition, as though Curtis had told a story about a mild blizzard that they had all lived through two months ago. Not a single person in the room was surprised by this story. When I mentioned Curtis's life-altering move in other settings throughout our travels in the United States, the same thing happened: no one raised an eyebrow. In fact, US teachers and students mainly seemed perplexed that I found the massage therapist's story noteworthy in the first place.

For a Canadian, such talk is baffling. A friend of mine recently joked that in Canada the successful five-season run of the American TV show *Breaking Bad* would have ended after episode 1, with Walter White returning to his classroom aware that he will not need to become a drug kingpin because he will be offered free health care for his stage-three lung cancer.

My interactions with Curtis, Steve, and Donna occurred in the first two days of fieldwork but echoed in my mind for months. They underlined differences between our societies, as well as the steep learning curve that I had in front of me.

Mats, Maps, and Territories

There is a lot of value in what American sociologist C. Wright Mills calls "the sociological imagination," which refers to a tendency to see people as enmeshed in and the products of much larger social forces and institutions. Of course, as I observed earlier, these forces influence us in ways that we do not generally notice. If we are fish, they create much of the water in which we swim. This is the main reason people who believe that they are radically free often do not seem to notice that they dress and decorate their homes in more or less the same ways as everyone else in their social circles.

What I found in my research is that the current mood within yogaland is generally non- and sometimes anti-sociological. When I try to make connections between anti-world yoga spaces and the larger political realities of the world, most of my fellow practitioners look at me as though I have just brought up mutual funds or crypto currency in a wedding speech.

To be clear, some practitioners are quite happy to talk about these social forces, but in general, the anti-worlds of yogaland are not designed to facilitate active, critical interrogation of this nature. That is not an indictment of yoga practitioners but an almost default orientation in our individualistic society. In fact, many journalists and scholars interested in postural yoga in the contemporary world tend to focus either on the ways that individuals use yoga to address specific micro (physical) concerns in their lives or on the ways that yogaland is influenced by macro (global) forces such as capitalism, colonialism, and sexism. We – researchers, journalists, practitioners – tend to neglect the meso (societal) level when we talk, write, teach, or think about yoga. That is, we tend to ignore that these particular yoga bodies are on mats in Kelowna, British Columbia, which is in Canada, or they are on mats in Killeen, Texas, which is in the United States.

The tendency to neglect the meso-level political dimensions of postural yoga – a tendency certainly evident in popular and scholarly writing about yoga – makes it hard to understand how its practice and meaning differ across societies and regions and why yoga became popular in the first place.[21] Without thinking about the extent to which yoga in New York reflects specifically New York (or East Coast) big-city considerations that would be irrelevant for practitioners in Victoria (or arguably even in Indianapolis), we miss something important.

This focus on the micro-individual (bodily) and the macro-political (ideological) vantage points also makes it hard for teachers and students like Tara, who are necessarily situated in a broader (meso) society, to get the most out of their practice. That is, postural yoga certainly responds, as advertised, to physical problems. Occasionally, there are considerations in yogaland of macro forces such as capitalism, colonialism, and patriarchy, but rarely do practitioners or scholars take seriously (enough) relatively meso-level forces such as race, class, ethnicity, and nationalism. This oversight is unfortunate since we come in contact with these forces when interacting with nationally specific (or state/province-specific) medical institutions, reparation and reconciliation movements, public schools, and military crises, among others. These interactions have a very significant impact on our day-to-day experiences as well as on the bodies (and minds) that we bring to the yoga studio.

Students and teachers often observe that yoga is ultimately about "the inward turn," as one participant said, referring to the power of yoga and meditation to cultivate a rich internal life that creates distance between ourselves and a heartless world that seems to impinge upon us. This claim is in keeping with much of what we know about the history of yoga from medieval South Asia to modern North America. Regardless of what this turn reveals, it occurs in particular bodies situated in particular times and societies, and that matters.

But maybe it does not matter as much as I had thought. Initially, I began my research with a focus on how distinctively Canadian and American approaches to health care, women's reproductive autonomy, and cultural diversity might impact the way that yoga is taught and experienced in these two countries. These differences are real, and they show up throughout this book. But in fact, what I found is that the contrast that seems to matter most is not between the United States and Canada in the narrow sense but between the world on and off the mat.[22]

"The map is not the territory."[23] Professors use this pithy declaration to underline the differences between the actual world (the territory) and the ways that we imagine the world (the map). The key lesson is that we orient ourselves in time and space through stories about the world that have been handed down to us by our religious and ethnic communities, families, nations, cultures, and peer groups. These accounts of the world, these maps, are necessarily partial and often grossly distorted. As we saw in the stories about Steve, Donna, and Curtis, one person's map often looks bizarre to another. The dilemma, of course, is that without maps, our world would be overwhelming. The goal of growing up, it seems to me, is to work continually to update the maps that we use as individuals and communities – to add newly discovered rivers, bike lanes, Indigenous burial sites, expanding suburbs, and earthquake fault lines.

For some North American yogis I met in this study and in other contexts, one might say that *the mat is the territory*. That is, what happens on these roughly 12 square feet of rubber speaks directly to all the struggles and strife that we can see in the world outside. For them, a yoga practice is inherently political. Yes, while on the mat, one should improve oneself mentally and physically, respect the teacher's instructions, and perform asanas in a careful, deliberate manner. But as a few teachers advocated, one should also be working to bring this improved self into right relations with the surrounding society.[24]

When I asked John, a teacher in Vancouver, whether his yoga classes were influenced by political considerations, he said,

[In the last several years,] I became more aware of my need to be an inclusive yoga teacher. And so today [in the class that I had just taken with him], I had you look down past the tip of your nose and relax your eyes. [I said,] "If it's relaxing for you to close your eyes, close your eyes." That [intervention comes] out of the reading I've done on trauma, on being Black in America, where you invite people. Because closing your eyes if you've been abused is not a safe place. [That] never occurred to me before.

He gestured to himself and laughed, drawing attention to his white-maleness as he explained,

I have all of the privilege! Like *all* of it! So I'm really lucky in that way, but I didn't have to deal with any of [that discrimination] growing up … And so I've really worked to educate myself in how I can be more inclusive as a yoga teacher. Like how I can, you know, just be, just be aware of the language I'm using. And I was already aware of the issues of the patriarchy and yoga but maybe less so the issues of the patriarchy and white rule in the West.

I observed that, despite having returned to Vancouver from Los Angeles several years ago, he had referred to the Black Lives Matter movement rather than to the reconciliation discussions occurring in Canada. He remarked, "Maybe that's because I lived in LA for so long," explaining that he had left Canada in 1997 when reconciliation with displaced and abused Indigenous people "wasn't an issue. I mean, obviously it was a huge issue, but it wasn't an issue we talked about." John also noted that if what he taught in yoga class "had not spun out into [a student's] life in some way, then I would think that I wasn't doing my job."

Although Indigenous political issues almost never arose without me introducing them into discussions, two Canadians did offer some relevant reflections.

Sandy, a senior student and teacher in Vancouver of Métis (French and Indigenous) ancestry, said, "I always start my class with the territorial acknowledgment. Always. For me it's not even a question. And this makes people sometimes uncomfortable. People are on their mat [expressing some concern over the acknowledgment], and I'm like, 'Well, get used to it because that's what happens in my class.'"

Helen, a recently trained teacher at a hot yoga studio in Toronto, noted that she tries to remind students of the importance of Indigenous reconciliation. "At the end of each class, I say collectively ..., 'Let's take this time to acknowledge our breath, because it's the only thing that's with us from the moment that we enter this planet to the moment that we leave it behind ... [Let's acknowledge] this land on which we practise and on which we play, and [also let's acknowledge] the roots of the yoga tradition that have followed us into our modern day.'"

Yet, for a clear majority of North American yogis I have met, the *mat is not the territory* insofar as their practice is either intentionally divorced from or only very obliquely connected with the outside world. For them, the studio anti-world is a "sacred" – students and teachers regularly used this term – respite from a chaotic and cruel world. Shanice, the owner and lead teacher of a studio in New York that caters mainly to African American students, said,

[Creating an escape is] why I have to have this space. Because who wants to talk about Trump? Who wants to talk about guns? Who wants to talk about *Roe versus Wade*? Who wants to talk about all [that]? I want people to come for ninety minutes and turn all that rhetoric off. And that's why I'm saying, "You sit in your shit. Sit here and let whatever needs to come up. Let it come up. Put your tears here, your blood here, your sweat here. Leave it all here." I [burn] sage. I clear it out. And then you go on out there [into the world] and be a rock star.

One teacher, Toni, contended,

I want my yoga room, for lack of a better word, to be open to everybody. And why does anyone need to know my opinion [about politics]? Because I stand for what yoga stands for, which is equal rights, which is the freedom of speech, which is, you know, all of these main issues, but I don't want to put it in the political context.

But it's very hot within the greater yoga community. I've had people attack me for not being more outwardly verbal in my social media about the Black Lives Matter [movement]. But if they just scratched beneath the surface, they would see that each and every one of my courses has a lot of content related to [social justice concerns]. I'm just not publicly out in that way. It's not my preferred stance in life to be creating any level of oppositional energy. I'm interested in the "yes and," in the middle path, and finding the ways that we can connect and evolve together ...

There's a lot of people in the yoga world who believe that you should be into politics if you're into yoga, that it's your civil duty to be into politics if you're into yoga, which, which I don't personally agree with ... And so then I really turned my focus inwardly ... The greatest form of activism is to clear up your own self, to clean your mind, to, you know, come to terms with who you are and how you are. And, you know, walk with integrity through life, as hard as that is sometimes.

When Kelly, a senior teacher in the vinyasa yoga community of Indianapolis, reflected on the social and political consequences of the overturning of the *Roe v. Wade* decision, she noted, "I felt just this heaviness, this collective heaviness. People are just like, 'Okay, this is life now.' [But] you know, [now that the pandemic has subsided and Trump is no longer president,] people are, I think, are starting to settle back into feeling okay. But the feeling of just the weight after all of that happened was very intense." When I asked whether practising yoga might address this heavy mood, she said, "I think yoga makes everything more tolerable. That's just my experience with it. [It allows people] to process, to feel, to just let yourself be in whatever you're in, you know?"

Her friend and fellow practitioner Martha entered the conversation and said,

I think it brings [up] emotions differently for everyone. Everyone has a connection to it in a different way, even if you're a man or a woman. [The reversal of the *Roe v. Wade* decision] means something for everybody. So I think [a yoga studio is] a safe space to show up even if just to move your body, not even have to think, you know what I mean? That's another thing – because sometimes you just want to go [to a teacher-led or a vinyasa class] to be told what to do, and, you know, that can help too.[25]

Conclusion

It is certainly worthwhile to raise critical questions about the ways that postural yoga communities can unintentionally strengthen the social forces that have mangled our bodies and brought our world to a political and environmental precipice. Although there are recent moves to welcome conversations about politics into yoga spaces, critics correctly observe that exposing and opposing these social forces have not been central concerns.

Nevertheless, yoga studios are carefully designed oases. The spaces are clean and quiet, with muted colours and Indic art, air tinged with incense, and rules that most people obey without needing to be reminded. In fact, studios entail a great many other entirely invisible design choices that reflect an owner's values and their interpretation of broad yogic principles. Toward the end of my fieldwork, I asked the owner of my own recently renovated studio to tell me about her design process. I had anticipated hearing about Indic imagery and perhaps her colour palette. However, what she said was far more interesting:

Well, we used "lotus" lights in the practice spaces that are CRI [colour rendering index] 95 and daylight quality, which gets sunlight quality into the skin, [and I installed] dimmers at select locations to set ambiance, [and we put high-carbon] Shungite powder into the black paint to ease EMF [electro-magnetic frequency], [and we chose] to use no VOC [volatile organic chemicals] paint and low off-gassing cork floors. The real wood we used has water-based finish, [and we installed] a water filtration system at the entrance of the water main to the unit, so every faucet and every shower has high-quality, filtered, no-chlorine water, along with replacing old pipes with PEX [cross-linked polyethylene pipes], which have no BPA [bisphenol A]. We have two high-quality HEPA [high-efficiency particulate absorbing] air purifiers that are both filters and humidifiers. And, of course, [we ensure] careful curation of the retail [offerings] so it is as local as possible and supports [asana] practice.

It struck me that although this owner (with a graduate degree in health science and decades of experience as a teacher) did not make explicit references to the many gods and gurus who appear on the walls or in statue form in her studio, she was nonetheless explaining how she had turned what sociologist Émile Durkheim might have called an ordinary (or "profane," as he would have said) space into a sacred or set-aside space. It seems to me that her design decisions were political in the sense that they reflected a thoughtful reimagination of this space such that it would be free of some of the worst aspects of an often toxic world.

More broadly, studios are alternatives to societies shaped by a neoliberal ideology that is both aggressive (in the sense of corroding the welfare state) and indifferent (in the sense of being uncaring about the consequences of limiting governmental involvement in our well-being). As Joyce, a senior teacher in the United States, noted, "I think there are a lot of people who get distressed by the political realities [of our world], and yoga helps them to deal with their stress and distress about it, and it helps them to be strong enough to be able to build a space in a way that's constructive instead of destructive."

Later in the book, I discuss the ways that the "body keeps the score," a reference to a massively popular book of the same name by Bessel van der

Kolk.[26] Clearly, people carry in their flesh and bones all manner of mental, emotional, spiritual, and physical distress. It is tempting but, in my view, ultimately unsatisfying to condemn studios that separate themselves deliberately or inadvertently from the political territories where their students, with their burdened bodies, are located. A more direct engagement with the gross or subtle forms of politics discussed in this chapter is always possible, but it is hardly surprising that such an approach is not very popular.[27]

Sometimes an opiate is a compassionate intervention that may offer people just enough peace of mind and relief of body that they can imagine another world. Whether one considers these imaginative acts to be political, spiritual, or religious in nature is another question, one that I address in the next chapter.

CHAPTER TWO

Religionish

Although my initial experiences in my shala (yoga studio) offered a way out or through the dark prognosis that my doctor had provided, I knew that it would take some time to soothe my furious joints. In order not to be distracted, I decided that I would just ignore any references to South Asian philosophy and religion that I might encounter at the Ashtanga shala. The fact that I thought that I could do so seems ridiculous in retrospect, but I was very motivated. My single-minded pursuit of what I thought would be a vaguely Indic form of physiotherapy ended after practice one morning as I was on my way to the change room.

"What I like is that yoga has nothing to do with religion," one of the teachers said in a conversation with a new student who was enthusing over her discovery of yoga.

The student seemed to understand the teacher's meaning and replied, "Right. Totally, I get it. It's so awesome." The conversation shifted to weekend plans.

I tried just to observe rather than to think about this comment, but I failed. It was a disorienting experience, so I continued to the change room, put on some fresh clothes, and packed up my gear. I had every intention of walking past the reception desk with a grateful nod and a soft thank you, as is the custom in most studios.

My very sensible plan was ruined by Shiva Nataraja, the God of the Dance. Bronze statues of Shiva are present in many studios; typically, they are about 10 inches tall. Shiva – one of the main divinities in the Hindu pantheon – is usually surrounded by a ring of fire and is dancing on the back of an infant. As I turned toward Mikki at the front desk, perfectly prepared for a soft exit, I noticed the ubiquitous Shiva for the first time on the shelf behind her head. I am not sure why I had not noticed it before; perhaps my efforts at compartmentalization had been working well. Until now.

I was pleased that instead of blurting something out, I pivoted slightly so that I could collect my thoughts and pretend to look at the shala's bookshelf. This choice simply added heat to the thought process underway in my mind since the only books there were the *Bhagavad Gita*; Edwin Bryant's *The Yoga Sutras of Patanjali* (2009); Guy Donahaye and Eddie Stern's *Guruji: A Portrait of Sri K. Pattabhi Jois through the Eyes of His Students* (2010); and Sharmila Desai and Anna Wise's *Yoga Sadhana for Mothers: Shared Experiences of Ashtanga Yoga, Pregnancy, Birth and Motherhood* (2014). When others had left the foyer and I had exhausted my abilities to look like someone who was not waiting for a conversation, I adopted the tone I use when asking innocuous questions.[1]

"Hey, Mikki. Great class," I began. "I hope this doesn't sound strange, and obviously you can feel free not to answer, but just now you told that woman with the lotus tattoo – "

"Lisa?"

"Right, Lisa. You said that yoga has nothing to do with religion. What did you mean?"

"Aren't you a religious studies professor?"

"Uhh, yeah, but I work on modern Western stuff, so I'm new to this. I don't have a correct answer in mind. Promise," I sort of lied.

"Well, it just isn't about religion. I mean, yoga's beyond all that."

"Okay, cool. I think I see what you mean. But it has roots in capital-R religions, right?"

"Sure. Long time ago, but it's not really tied to them anymore, which is why no one here talks about Hinduism or pujas or the Buddha or anything like that."

"Fair enough. But I mean, what happens here is also not *not* religious, right?"

"Well, I guess I'd say it's not."

"Hang on." A small part of my mind could sense that I was crossing a threshold, but I stuffed this thought into a mental cubbyhole, and then I said, "So what I mean is that teachers and senior students call the lineage bosses guru, guruji, or even paramaguru. At led classes, we stand together, bow our heads, and recite a Sanskrit invocation that dates back to the fourteenth century and includes references to gods, sages, mythical creatures, and other theological concepts. Not everyone does the chant, but literally everyone stands and bows. Also, sometimes when I arrive in the morning, the sound of 'om' is playing on a speaker in the foyer. I'm completely fine with this, but, I mean – "

"Okay, okay, I see. Yes. Uhhhhmmm," Mikki said, probably wondering if the shala should tighten up its membership rules.

"And on top of that," I continued, "throughout the shala there are statues of Ganesh, Shiva, and Patanjali, draped in prayer beads with flowers at their feet, hanging bronze medallions of the 'om' symbol, a framed actual leaf supposedly from the tree under which the Buddha sat when he was enlightened about 2,500 years ago. Teachers usually use Sanskrit names for asanas even if that is all the Sanskrit they know.[2] Oh yeah, and we don't practise on 'moon days,' which I guess are both about the phases of the moon but also Indian astrology. This is not a complete list, but – "

"Seriously?"

We both laughed.

"Okay, okay, I know – sorry, occupational hazard. The list is pretty complete, I guess. Believe it or not, there's a lot of debate in my world about the definition of 'religion,' and I won't bore you with that, but – "

"God, thanks. Please don't," she said with a wink and a wide grin.

"Ha! No problem. But it's interesting that I bet everyone here would say what you just said, which is that this place has nothing to do with religion. But that list I gave you just off the top of my head includes a lot of capital-R religion stuff."

"Well, okay, hmmm. But again, I guess what I really mean is that it is spiritual, not religious."

"Ha! Now we've jumped from the frying pan into the fire."

One would be less likely to have the same conversation with yoga teachers and students in more fitness-oriented spaces such as GoodLife Fitness, the YMCA, BeFitNYC, Orangetheory, or Equinox. Mind you, even in these settings, one can detect *religionish* features in the idea of setting an intention, breathing together, and centring, not to mention the soft lighting or the teacher's (often vaguely Indic) clothing, jewelry, tattoos, and choice of music. It is not unusual even at the end of a fitness-oriented yoga class in a corporate gym setting to see people with no grasp of Sanskrit at all sit up from shavasana (corpse pose; see figure 2.1), bow slightly toward the teacher, and say a soft namaste, which means "a bow to you," although it is sometimes translated as "that within me which is also within you, greets you."

Most of the teachers and students with whom we talked for the project agree with Mikki: yoga is spiritual but not religious. It seems to me that in order to understand postural yoga in North America, we need to understand what people mean by that. To be clear, I am not interested in whether postural yoga is *actually* spiritual rather than religious, both religious and spiritual, or entirely religious. I am just curious about why people speak, think, and act as they do.

After all, the claims that "Yoga is spiritual" and that "Yoga is not religious" might seem straightforward, but in fact their meanings are no more self-evident than the statements "unemployment is a problem," "the United States is a beacon of freedom," or "Canada is the home of peace, order, and good government." All of these claims are pregnant with other meanings and assumptions.[3] Before we reflect on why yoga is so often framed as spiritual rather than religious, a quick trip to some yoga studios is in order.

When you register for your first class at a new studio, you will usually be asked to provide some basic details (e.g., name, address, and billing information) and to sign a waiver that protects the studio in case you are accidentally injured. In addition, you will often be asked whether you have had any previous yoga experience and, if so, what kind (e.g., vinyasa, Ashtanga, Iyengar, or hot). This intake process helps teachers to understand students' needs and preconceptions about yoga. You (almost certainly) will not be asked about your religion.

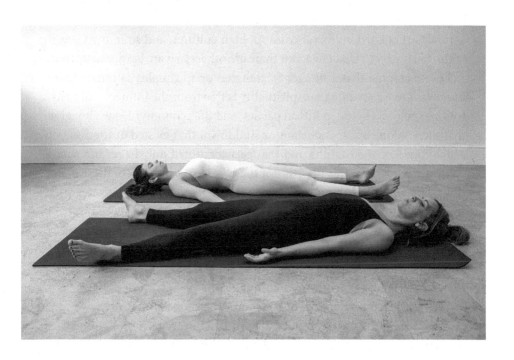

Figure 2.1
Shavasana (corpse pose)

Whenever one thinks or talks about religion and spirituality, it is worthwhile to do an inventory about what one already knows and thinks (or what one thinks one knows). Although I cannot know what prior commitments readers bring to this book, I should note that over roughly the past thirty years, key thinkers have called into question some of the often hidden preconceptions that scholars and laypeople have about these core concepts.[4]

Do we assume, for example, that there is one religious or spiritual path (e.g., Christianity) that is true, and all others are deviations? This assumption is rarely articulated in liberal cosmopolitan cultures, and so in my view, it is also fairly easy to challenge. But there are others that are harder to uproot.

Do we assume that a hunger for religion or spirituality is innate to all humans? Do we assume that spirituality is free from the influence of institutions such as religion, political parties, and the economy? Do we imagine that there is one authentic Islam or Buddhism that existed at the time of Muhammad or the Buddha and that gets corrupted only in certain social contexts? Obviously, this book is not the place to discuss any of these questions. Nonetheless, I think that it is useful to bear in mind that categories such as religion, spirituality, sacred, secular, and so forth are used in particular ways for particular ends – usually to solve certain problems or to organize certain communities. That is as true when we talk about "the separation of church and state" in the United States as it is when we talk about Canada's "secular form of multiculturalism."[5]

Yet these terms do not exist in a vacuum. Such concepts are not any more natural than terms such as beauty, art, truth, wife, home, nation, or justice. Our culture seems to have adjusted reasonably well to critiques of words such as beauty and wife by feminists and to critiques of words such as justice and truth by lawyers and activists. We might say that a person, building, or painting is beautiful, but we often add or assume that it is understood that we mean "according to the standards of such and such a time and place." Similarly, it is common to assume that different cultures, and even different individuals within the same culture, may embrace very different understandings of justice.

We have benefited tremendously by expanding our understandings of the meaning(s) of concepts such as beauty, gender, and justice. But many people still speak of religion, the sacred, spirituality, and the secular as though these were not negotiable metaphors but rather unproblematic labels, such as "the parsnip" or "the cat." In my view, the experiences, objects, or groups that we describe as religious, sacred, and spiritual should be understood to be just as evolving, culturally particular, and sometimes idiosyncratic as the experiences, objects, and groups that we describe as beautiful, feminine, just, and so on.

In this chapter, I tease apart the claim that yoga is spiritual but not religious in an effort to see what kinds of broader forces in and around yogaland make such an assertion possible (or appealing). In the process, I think that it becomes clear both that the distinction is artificial and that the distinction produces its own absurdities when looked at carefully enough. However, elsewhere in the book, I use the categories of religion, spirituality, and so on as they are used in yogaland, without using scare quotes or other means to demonstrate these terms' socially constructed nature. I take this approach for the sake of expediency since a thorough analysis of these terms is beyond this chapter, but readers are encouraged to imagine scare quotes around these words.

I mentioned the formal invocation that one hears at an Ashtanga yoga studio; a similar invocation is also used in many Iyengar contexts.[6] Indeed, almost all yoga classes that I have attended begin with ritualized gestures, such as a collective "om," synchronized breathing, or setting an intention, all of which are coordinated by a teacher and hallowed by weighty silence. I focus on the Ashtanga invocation not just because I have heard or intoned it many hundred times over the years – and had to perform it myself in order to pass the teacher-training course that I took – but also because it is indicative of some broader patterns. It is also a moment when what I think of as the *religionish* elements of a serious yoga practice might be evident.

The Sanskrit shlokas (verses) being chanted evoke a world that is both broadly Indic and somewhat more specifically "Hindu," to use a word that did not come into wide circulation until the late-modern period when scholarship on nation building and Orientalism combined to promote the idea that everyone belongs to one or another of the "world religions." The chant connects the ancient and the modern too, at least in the sense that it has roots in the distant past but in its present form was established – one might say canonized – by Tirumalai Krishnamacharya in the twentieth century. The invocation is recited at the beginning of led Ashtanga classes (where there is one teacher leading everyone through the same series of postures) and also at many Mysore-style classes (where students work independently through the series while teachers move about the room offering advice, adjustments, and new postures).

Before the chanting begins, a teacher enters the room and says something like, "Come to samasthiti" (equal standing posture). In the many Ashtanga settings in which I have practised since 2013, students stop whatever else they might have been doing and stand at the front of their mat attentively, hands in prayer position in front of their chests, heads slightly bowed, and eyes closed, as they silently wait for the teacher to speak. Often, when the class includes beginners, the teacher is likely to say something along the lines of, "This is just a way to thank our teachers. You can feel free to hum along or say nothing."

What then follows is the Ashtanga invocation, offered in either a call-and-response or unison format, which I present here phonetically:

Om
Vande Gurunam Charanaravinde
Sandarshita Svatma Sukava Bodhe
Nih Sreyase Jangalikayamane
Samsara Halahala Mohashantyai

Abahu Purushakaram
Shankhacakrsi Dharinam
Sahasra Sirasam Svetam
Pranamami Patanjalim
Om

Here is a translation of the original Sanskrit:

Om

I bow to the lotus feet of the Gurus
The awakening happiness of one's own Self revealed,

Beyond better, acting like the Jungle Physician,
Pacifying delusion, the poison of Samsara.

Taking the form of a man to the shoulders,
Holding a conch, a discus, and a sword,
One thousand heads white,
To Patanjali, I salute.

Om[7]

I do not think that it would be very useful to do a lengthy close reading of this invocation since I use it mainly as an entry point to thinking about why and how religion is bracketed in favour of spirituality. Nonetheless, it is helpful to observe the tension between the actual chant and the reassurance that I have heard perhaps a hundred times now ("This is just a way to thank our teachers"). The father of modern yoga, Tirumalai Krishnamacharya, crafted the invocation in the twentieth century, but the first verse comes from the *Yoga Taravali*, a fourteenth-century poem attributed to Adi Shankara, who was a scholar, renunciant, mystic, and for some, avatar of the Lord Shiva. The second verse is of unknown provenance but arguably much older than the first.

Readers will notice first that asanas are not mentioned specifically; instead, the emphasis is on Indian theology and mythology: samsara (the cycle of birth, death, and rebirth), pure being, gods, and avatars.[8] There are rich mythological threads connecting samsara, the "lotus feet of the Gurus," "one's own Self revealed," and the reference to Patanjali, who has assumed the form of a man but is also possibly an avatar of Adishesha (sometimes known as Ananta Shesha), a primordial Indic god.

Second, readers will observe that the teachers being mentioned are ancient personages imbued with more-than-human attributes rather than the twentieth-century asana masters: Krishnamacharya, Pattabhi Jois, B.K.S. Iyengar, and T.K.V. Desikachar, among others. Very few people in these studios would read or understand spoken Sanskrit. One senior Iyengar student in Toronto said, "We do a chant as well at the beginning of many classes. We say it, but I don't think anybody knows what they're saying." I suspect that if students were more aware of what they were saying, questions might arise about what it would mean for someone in 2023 Indianapolis or Halifax to thank a being with thousands of white heads.

In other words, the statement "This is just a way to thank our teachers" is a basically true but not entirely honest representation of the invocation. I confess that I resist this observation since I enjoy the invocation and respect the teachers who lead it. When my undergraduate students visit my shala and the teachers offer the standard account of the invocation, I know that I will need to answer some questions the next time that the undergraduate class meets. After all, in my university course on yoga, I spend a class talking about the invocation, so the students are often confused by the breezy explanation that they hear at the shala.

In a discussion period in our class, a smart Catholic student remarked, "I guess it would be like saying that the Apostles' Creed is just a way to say Jesus is also God."

I felt a bit defensive and replied, "Sort of, though the other claim that is often made, or assumed, in yoga spaces, is that the meaning of the invocation transcends the literal or grammatical meaning of the sentences. The fact that people don't understand the actual Sanskrit words or sentences they are chanting is not a huge problem because the actual meaning and purpose of the chant is conveyed through the spirit, the music, or the magic, of the sound itself. Also, chanting beside other people doesn't just unify the group, it constitutes it – remember talking about Émile Durkheim last class? – and so the meaning arises through a kind of unspoken consensus."

The student raised his eyebrows. "I guess that makes sense, but it sounds a lot like what was going on in Catholic churches a hundred years ago when people were still doing the singing, praying, and all that in Latin."

In retrospect, I think that I had wanted what happens in the shala to be different from what happens in obviously religious settings where mysterious higher powers are invoked and groups are bound together through ritualized actions and sacralized language, but of course, it is not.

"Right, well put," I replied to the clever student.

Virtually all of the teachers who offer newcomers this generic reassurance about teacher thanking have been through the same workshops and Yoga Alliance–approved teacher-training program that I went through, and some have received far more training than I have.[9] As a result, they know quite well the more complicated story behind the chants.

But clearly there is a difference between knowing about the backstory of the invocation and being able to present this knowledge as a digestible morsel of information. However, even before a teacher considered how or whether to convey the invocation's context to students, they would need to consider what it could possibly mean for them – a middle-class, white, female, Baptist dentist and yoga instructor from Atlanta, for example – to thank avatars for eliminating the "poison of Samsara."

In my first few years at the shala, it was nearly impossible for me to chant without thinking about the core claims in the sentences being uttered. When I tried to join the others in the room, the words stuck in my throat, so I hummed along or just mentally checked out. But in the past several years, things have changed. Now, I quite appreciate the chant and no longer think about the line-by-line English translations that my mind used to superimpose over top of what I was saying in Sanskrit.

In some sense, doing so is a compromise, perhaps even a capitulation to a set of ideas and practices that originate in or bear a strong family resemblance to religion. Perhaps it just means that I have become – despite my best efforts – a normal member of a normal religionish group, with some degree of the conformity that this membership entails. Nonetheless, it seems to me that most of my fellow teachers and students are content to bracket the esoteric philosophical elements of the invocations heard in studios across yogaland. Instead, their focus is on the feelings that the invocation allows – both the sense of solidarity with others in the room and the ineffable feeling of wholeness that the experience occasions in their bodies.

I encountered the invocation in Victoria at my first "half primary" led class one Friday evening in February 2014. In the Ashtanga subculture, a "led" class is what most people imagine by a normal yoga class: one teacher, many students, the latter all moving in a manner determined by the former. The implied contrast in this community is between "led" and "Mysore" classes, the latter referring to the open format described earlier.

I had been avoiding the half primary because it is quite advanced, and I really enjoyed the fairly light "community classes" that I had taken for the previous three months. I was encouraged by my teachers, Annie and Jack, to try "the half," although I was worried that I would not be able to keep up with the other students (many of whom were twenty years younger). Still, Annie and Jack assured me that I was ready for the Friday evening half primary.

So, after quietly slipping into the dark back corner of the practice room, I followed the lead of the teacher and my fellow students and took my place standing in samasthiti at the front of my mat. The teacher began the class by introducing the chant to the eighteen students in the room with the conventional "This is just a way to thank our teachers" disclaimer, encouraging people to remain silent if they were so inclined.

For a then forty-six-year-old newcomer with unfaithful joints, the half primary has the same relationship to the community classes as a half marathon has to a leisurely jog. A teacher once explained that asana practice ought to be seen as a breathing practice accompanied by bodily postures. Fair enough, to an extent. Once the physical postures became familiar to me, and once I understood how to pair them with deep measured breathing, I became able – as have others, according to their own stories – to "sink into" my practice and to experience sublime moments that combine a strange sense of tremendous lightness and profound rootedness. Now, on good days, I experience a unique sense of being on my mat in my body (and definitively nowhere else) yet simultaneously and intractably connected to some much larger order (and thus everywhere else). This sensation certainly does not arise every time I practice, and the feeling does not last very long, but I do not think I would continue my practice without knowing that the sensation might occur. My knees were tamed in a matter of a few months, but I suppose I have remained for the combination of spiritual transformation and social engagement – the traces of which readers will see throughout this book.

In hot yoga settings, the room is preheated to between roughly 36 and 40 degrees Celsius (97 and 105 degrees Fahrenheit), but Ashtanga and Iyengar rooms begin at about room temperature. Nevertheless, I was not just fatigued and wet at the end of my first half primary when the class entered shavasana but also simply relieved that I had not lost consciousness.

That Friday evening as I drove home, I was lost in a reverie caused by the rhythmic communal breathing, the humidity and heat generated entirely by the nineteen minimally clad people in the room, and the gravitas in the teacher's voice as he delivered the invocation, counted breaths, and announced each asana in Sanskrit. However, in addition to the physical difficulty of the class, there were also psychological, intellectual, and ideological challenges. Between my mixed-race family history and my admiration for critics such as Talal Asad, Edward Said, Saba Mahmood, and Noam Chomsky, I found myself simultaneously enthralled and slightly distressed by this experience.

I have a deep aversion to saying things that I (possibly) do not believe and in a language that I (certainly) do not understand, especially when this language is (distantly) related to a heritage from which my family alienated itself through indentured labour migration from India over a century ago. So I stayed silent throughout the invocation and watched and listened as the rest of the class – all white people, as far as I could tell – followed the teacher's lead.

"How was it?" my partner asked when I returned from the shala that night. I paused for an unusually long time.

"Hello?" she nudged with her voice from the other room.

"Uhhh. I don't know. I don't have words to describe what just happened. It was weird, I guess? And extraordinary? And weird? And I need to think more about it all. I sort of think I love it, though?" An hour later, showered, fed, and more or less level-headed, I entered my home office and assured myself that Googling the chant's history and meanings reflected my innocent curiosity. (The idea that this practice might also become the centre not just of my research life but also of my religious or spiritual life within the next few years was almost inconceivable at this point.)

The next time that I saw Jack, my teacher and the studio co-owner, I asked whether he thought that it might be worthwhile to post the chants in Sanskrit and English in the change rooms in case students might like to see what they are hearing or saying. I have had so many versions of this discussion with so many teachers and advanced students over the years (and in spaces dedicated to so many different forms of yoga) that a composite conversation should convey what transpires almost every time.

"Hey, Jack, so I wonder – what would you think about me printing out translations of the opening and closing chants and putting them in the change rooms?"

I was not prepared for the blank look that this sincere, if somewhat naive, question would elicit not just from Jack but also from everyone else to whom I posed it over the next several years.

"Well, that's interesting, but why?" He shrank into his chair a little when he asked this question.

"I guess I wonder if people might like to connect their asana practice to Patanjali, the idea of the jungle physician, the snake god, samsara, and so on?"

"Yeah, maybe, but couldn't they just Google it like you did?"

"Sure, they could. But isn't it always better for people to have more rather than less knowledge about what they're doing and saying?"

"Interesting. I just wonder if it might mess with a person's experience if they got too bogged down in the details. I mean, we talk about these kinds of things when we do workshops."

He had a good point, and I was trying hard not to argue. Nonetheless, I argued, "Right. Yeah, but workshops happen once or twice a year, and lots of people who practise a couple times a week wouldn't take them."

"Okay, but most people do the chant without knowing what it means, and those who don't want to do it, don't do it. From time to time, someone asks me about it, and I'm happy to answer, but hardly anyone ever asks. People tell me they love the chanting, so obviously our approach is kind of working. Basically, people don't seem that fussed about it. Except the religious studies professors," he said, at which point we both broke into laughter.

Regardless of whether I posed the idea in Ashtanga or other settings, the response to the idea of posting translations was almost always the same: *interesting idea; not going to do it.*

This issue reminded me of the decision of the Roman Catholic Church (following the Second Vatican Council in the 1960s) to switch from Latin to the ordinary languages spoken by parishioners. Traditionalists complained that to lose Latin would make the church too rational, too transactional – too Protestant, even. However, the difference between that context and the one that interests me here is that it was the Catholic Church itself that was trying to diminish Latin in order to make itself more accessible and modern. Eventually – to make a long story short – most Catholics saw the underlying logic of a shift toward greater transparency in their liturgy.

By contrast, almost no one we met in yogaland seemed very skeptical of the Sanskrit invocations one hears intoned in Ashtanga, Iyengar, and other settings. For reasons that I tease out in this book, studios are set-apart spaces, and different rules apply there. I am not entirely convinced that there is anything unique about claims or sounds made in Sanskrit – compared with, say, Dutch or Bulgarian – but many practitioners clearly felt that there is something magical about these oral (and aural) rituals. Joanne, an Iyengar teacher in Canada, contended that invocations had the effect of differentiating yoga from aerobics: "I think many studios like mine and like yours have kind of found the sweet spot. There's a little bit of references to Sanskrit, to India, to ancient Indic concepts, but not too much so that people don't feel like it's being like imposed on them, and they're being required to be Hindu or Buddhist or something like that. But it's enough that you feel like you're not just in a stretching class. You're not just in an aerobics class."

Either a balance has been struck, or for some other reason, people overlook the fact that they do not know any of the stories about the gods that are all over both the studio and the history and theology of the chant or what happened to the Buddha under the tree from which the framed leaf fell. This reliance on references to the gods is quite interesting given that practitioners have confidence that a tall wall of separation exists between their yoga practice and religion.

Yoga is spiritual but not religious.

This claim seems strange only when one notices that the same person who insists that their yoga practice has nothing to do with religion also spends ninety minutes, often several times each week, in a room decorated with Hindu deities, making shapes sometimes named for Indic sages and divinities, participating in a hierarchical guru-shishya (student) relationship with their teachers (to be discussed in chapter 5), hearing references to a revered ancient text often said to be composed by an avatar, and chanting in a language that they neither read nor speak – one that is spoken by under 1 per cent of Indians, most of whom are Brahmins.

People are often not at all troubled by intellectual tensions that we think might – or, truth be told, probably ought to – create some mental friction.

Outside of brief awkward moments in an interview, very few people seem to think about what many outsiders would recognize as the straightforwardly religious features of these spaces. After talking with so many teachers and students about the claim that yoga is spiritual but not religious, I can make four observations that may help to explain not just the religionish aspects of yogaland but perhaps also the ways that the border between spirituality and religion is created and policed.

First, in most liberal democracies, institutional religion is in decline and a source of unease. Once a feature of one's selfhood that for centuries would have been considered inalienable and even worth dying for, formal religious identification and activity have become increasingly optional, especially among younger cosmopolitans.

The British sociologist Linda Woodhead notes what has become almost obvious, namely that whereas Christian assumptions, tastes, and values were once found throughout Western societies and imaginations, people are now freer than ever to espouse fragments (or none) of these ideas and practices.[10] Clearly, the decline in both the popularity and prestige of religion[11] was accelerated by the scandals associated with clergy sexual abuse, church complicity in the assimilation project of First Nations residential schools (in Canada), the role of some churches in the uptick of right-wing populism (in the United States), and the sense that on issues related to sexuality, many churches were obstacles to the increasingly liberal, egalitarian, and secular culture.

My colleagues and I argue about the timeline and precise causes of secularization and about the relationship between secularization and the vested interests of the liberal elite who often celebrate it. We generally agree, however, not only that the term "secular" connotes a state of being in which religion recedes from the public arena and from personal lives over time but also that the conventional large expressions of institutional religion are in jeopardy in most Western liberal democracies. Major Christian institutions are seeing the most dramatic declines, but other communities are also struggling or are probably about to.[12] The general pattern that we can observe is that loyalty to conventional religious (especially Christian) institutions and identities is in decline in much of North America and in freefall in some places.[13]

What is important for our purposes is simply that the yoga students and teachers we interviewed clearly have stolid, conservative, androcentric religion in mind when they say that yoga has nothing to do with religion. They may recognize that there is an appetite for some of the things that we used to describe as religion/religious, but it is increasingly the case that people refer to these experiences, groups, leaders, books, events, and movements as spiritual. A common response came from Jamie, an authorized teacher in the Ashtanga community, who said: "I mean, I would categorize myself as a deeply spiritual person. I have a generic dislike for organized religion." So it is the case not just that organized religion is in decline but also that it is the cause of unease for many people.

Indeed, many teachers and senior students we met admitted that they are very careful to avoid explicit use of any language that people might interpret as religious or spiritual. Some even avoid using Sanskrit invocations altogether. John, a former Anusara teacher in Vancouver, noted, "I'll just even leave out the Sanskrit because I don't want to turn them off. I mean I want them to buy into what I'm offering. And so in that sense, you kind of secularize the Sanskrit teaching." Shanice, one of the few African American studio owners in New York, noted,

> And you know, the religious part for me, and I have to be really honest, is that I don't really delve into it because a lot of Black people won't do that. They won't, if it's too heavy in religion, they will not. I mean, I don't want to put the, the spin of religion on it too much. I like to say "spirituality" … So if I have an old Trinidadian woman, I'm not going to say "om" five times in my class. I might say it once because I still have to honour who I am and the truth. But like, yeah. I'm just very mindful of that.[14]

Clearly, all language that might even allude to religion is potentially problematic. As Karen, a former leader in the Los Angeles yoga scene, remarked, "I try to use the most simple language because I think that that's where I can reach more people. If I start to use, you know, religious language or even spiritual language, sometimes it turns people off." Kim, a hot yoga teacher in the United States, observed,

> I think someone who's not spiritual or doesn't believe in God could come and practise yoga and benefit hugely. And they could never

believe in God. They could never believe in anything spiritual. But they might learn to calm their mind just by stilling it and releasing whatever tension has been in their mind for, for years. But there's a lot of people I run into [in California] and who are so disillusioned by anything that's religious, by anything that's even spiritual, [because] I think [for them] spirituality has turned into something that's New Agey.

Nevertheless, religious and spiritual ideas still influence their teaching. "Most people come here to get fit," one senior Los Angeles Ashtanga teacher said. Laura knows that she has to deliver these sorts of results, but little by little she introduces spiritual dimensions into the practice by using the Sanskrit names of the asanas and by gradually introducing philosophical concepts such as karma (cause and effect), moksha (liberation), and samadhi (meditative absorption) into her explanations of the purpose of asana practice. "It's totally a bait and switch," she admitted, with a laugh.[15]

Second, the ways that people talk about yoga tell us something about the broader society. I do not think that it is very worthwhile to insist that incense, asana names, mala (garland) beads, pranayama (breath work) practices, the unison chanting of "om," or talk of chakras (energy centres) and nadis (energy channels) ought to be described or experienced as religious or spiritual. I do not have a horse in that proverbial race. The fact is that virtually no one we met in the project, and no one I have met during over a decade as a practitioner, explicitly connected these objects or practices with religion in any conventional or orthodox sense.

The fact that there is reticence to use religious or even quasi-religious language to talk about yoga and a preference for other terms – such as wellness, spirituality, and philosophy – tells us something about our existing options for talking about selves and transcendence. This trend is also reflected in the rise and power of what the sociologist Christian Smith calls "therapeutic individualism." In his study of the religious and spiritual life of younger Americans, he notes that therapeutic individualists

seek out religious and spiritual practices, feelings, and experiences that satisfy their own subjectively defined needs and wants. Faith and spirituality become centered less around a God believed in and God's claims on lives, and more around the believing (or perhaps even unbelieving) self and its personal realization and happiness. The very idea and language of "spirituality," originally grounded in the self-disciplining faith practices of religious believers, including ascetics and monks, then becomes detached from its moorings in historical religious traditions and redefined in terms of subjective self-fulfillment.[16]

The emergence of therapeutic individualism as a kind of default ethos for many people in our societies has profound and mostly negative implications for conventional religious communities.[17] Such an ethos is, almost by definition, hostile or at best indifferent to leaders, norms, and institutions that restrict autonomy or that might inspire shame. It is not an accident, then, that many sociologists and anthropologists of religion contend that the most interesting examples of contemporary North American spirituality come from communities, movements, and events well outside of conventional religious contexts.[18] Yoga spaces are, for many of us, the sites par excellence of these innovations.

It is important to note that the form of individualism that Smith describes is consistent with the dominant economic and political realities of our time. Neoliberalism encourages – indeed, perhaps requires – people to determine their own worldviews, serving themselves from a vast philosophical buffet, more and more unfettered by the judgments of society or a religious community. Yet when one detaches Indic ideas and practices – such as statues, invocations, and physical practices – from what Smith would call their religious "moorings," it is easy to disregard the troublesome aspects of Indic traditions to which one would normally object, such as ethnocentrism, casteism, the exclusion of women from certain leadership roles, and the conflation of religion and politics (as we see in Hindutva parties in India).[19]

The gap between the appreciation of India that many yoga teachers and students express and their awareness of its social and political realities is sometimes alarming. In a previous study, I examined a major and ultimately unsuccessful Canadian event planned to mark the inaugural International Day of Yoga in 2015.[20] When I looked at the vociferous public resistance to the event, it turned out that almost none of it had to do with the ways that Prime Minister Narendra Modi used this international campaign to boost his own national political ambitions and to distract global attention from his government's shortcomings. Why? People who weighed in on the Canadian event – including social justice activists and serious yoga students – were focused on local (Vancouver) concerns and had no interest in, and I suspect little awareness of, the political realities of India.

Although therapeutic individualism allows people to bracket the political problems evident in India, there are what we might think of as insider or spiritual dilemmas too. That is, the detachment or decoupling of the symbols of Indic practices from their deeper religious roots means that the transformative political implications of these symbols can be neutralized. It is in the interest of the neoliberal economic and political order that we defang any objectives (e.g., samadhi), texts (e.g., the *Bhagavad Gita* and the *Yoga Sutras*), and traditions (e.g., asceticism) that could offer us alternatives to the competitive, avaricious, individualistic society in which we find ourselves. I do not mean to suggest that these texts or traditions were primarily geared toward social justice; I doubt that such a case could be made convincingly. Rather – and I realize that this claim is common among insiders – yogic practices, including asanas, might be considered revolutionary simply by helping us to see clearly how awash we all are in avidya (ignorance of reality) and how attached we all are to our possessions, prestige, and samskaras (patterns of thought based on memories). Through this kind of awakening, at least in theory, we *could* gain the capacity to make different decisions about both our own lives and, at least potentially, our shared lives.

We live in a society where the marketplace is not just an expedient context in which to exchange resources for goods and services. Rather, we live in what the economist Karl Polanyi called a "market society" where all "social relations are embedded in the economic system."[21] How, then, might postural yoga fit into a society where the market is the social fact toward which all other institutions must point? If Smith is right about therapeutic individualism, then "subjective self-fulfillment" is the key personal driver of our lives. As a result, it is no wonder that since the flourishing of asana practice in the late 1980s, its main consumers have been the same ones whose classes we joined, the same ones we interviewed, and the same ones who responded to our survey – namely authenticity-seeking North Americans who feel increasingly untethered to their religious or familial heritage.

Third, in yogaland we see plenty of evidence of Orientalism. In his ground-breaking book *Orientalism* (1978), Edward Said outlined the ways that the West has romanticized and sometimes infantilized the "Orient." The European scholars, businesspeople, and politicians who took an interest in Asia over several centuries did so for a variety of reasons beyond simply the wealth that they could amass from theft, indentured labour, and asymmetrical trade relationships.[22] One of the main benefits of popularizing the idea of the East as a magical, mystical, feminine, traditional, and inscrutable place was that it helped Europeans, and more recently North Americans, to define themselves as rational, practical, scientific, modern, and masculine peoples over and against an impersonal cultural and geographical "other."

Readers familiar with the arrival of the East India Company in India in the early seventeenth century and with the forms of subservience to the British Crown that followed should expect this complicated history to be reflected in all South Asian cultural products – from yoga to Bollywood to spiritual tourism.[23] The connection between India's imperial past and yogaland's individualistic present can be both amusing and aggravating.

Norm, an Ashtanga teacher in the United States, noted how different yoga is in Asia, where he had lived and trained. "In the East, [yoga is] just something you do every day. Like it's just *there*. It's, it's a whole part of you. Spirituality is a part of you. It's not something external from you," as it is in the West.

A vinyasa flow teacher from Indianapolis who had trained in Rishikesh for many months noted, "Yoga was so unaffected in India. It's just, it's simple. The commands are simple. The postures are simple. The instruction is simple. This *[mimicking a posture]* is the thing, and you do it, and you breathe in and out, and it's done." Such images of India and yoga are certainly benevolent, although also perhaps just a little patronizing – an unintended echo of the ways that colonial administrators framed the residents of the territories they controlled as rather simple.

I confess that I grind my teeth a little whenever I hear North American teachers or fellow students wax poetic about India and its ineffable, inimitable, colourful, mystical, exquisite spiritual richness. Such comments are certainly well intended and – to be very clear – not exactly untrue. I understand what they mean, and I do not entirely disagree with them, but when the same North Americans are asked about the misogyny, air pollution, Is-lamophobia, Hindu nationalism, hunger, government corruption, and squelching of academic and press freedom that are also part of Indian life, many practitioners just shrug their shoulders and raise their eyebrows, re-fusing to articulate an opinion. Why? Here, I speculate that the fondness for India grows out of a need for some other society to symbolize a simpler time and to offer an affordable place for Westerners to reimagine themselves, much as Elizabeth Gilbert did in *Eat, Pray, Love* (2006).[24]

When Krishnamacharya revived and systematized hatha[25] yoga in the twentieth century, it was in part an act of resistance against the caricature of Indian men as weak, simple, and undisciplined.[26] Although he is credited with many innovations, the yoga that he and his students espoused relied on decidedly *religious* assumptions, philosophical schools of thought, rituals, language, and lines of authority. Nonetheless, thanks in part to Swami Vive-kananda's evangelism, the yoga(s) that arrived in the West in the twentieth century came wrapped in the pages of the *Yoga Sutras*.

According to Vivekananda, who did not in fact emphasize asanas, as well as to Swami Kuvalayananda, Krishnamacharya, and many other teachers in contemporary yogaland, asanas are a means of training the body – all bodies, from all religions and spiritual orientations – so that one can meditate more effectively. This training makes it more likely that one will experience both samadhi (meditative absorption) and kaivalya (solitude and liberation). In this sense, we could say that the yogic traditions inspired by Krishnama-charya, Vivekananda, and others are also consistent with the way that many people in the West today use the term "spiritual."[27] The transformation of well-moored religious (or religionish) terms and objectives into increasingly unmoored spiritual interests certainly reflects an effort to tame and con-strain religion in the modern era. However, this shift is not merely an example of the spread of secularism or therapeutic individualism mentioned earlier. It is also the case that the centrality of these now spiritualized and increasingly amorphous ideas and practices in yogaland also demonstrates that (even admittedly well-intended) Orientalist fantasies about Asia and Asian religious practices and concepts continue to flourish.

Fourth, students and teachers have variable levels of knowledge about their practice. It is common to describe postural yoga as spiritual but not religious yet to be unsure about what the "religious" aspects of yoga might be. That is not surprising. After all, postural yoga arrived in North America decades before the Internet increased our easy access to sound information about South Asian practices and ideas.

Modern postural yoga has thrived in urban centres among elites and hippies who often frame India in a romantic manner. Not long after it took root here – it arrived as early as 1893 but began to expand rapidly in the 1960s – asana practice was, as well, quickly taken up by entertainers and fitness adepts who were interested in yoga as beauty and stress-management regimes and who had neither the time nor the inclination to learn about yoga's other dimensions (not to mention Sanskrit).[28] Given that yoga has spread throughout Western societies in over just a few decades, whereas the practice developed over more than a thousand years in South Asia, it was inevitable that the recent adopters in North America would not be familiar with its long history and many facets.

I am reminded of a colleague of mine, Jim, who became passionate about Buddhism in his twenties by surreptitiously reading Alan Watts's books in his closet. A few years later, he left his home in Ontario to join a large monastery in Japan, where he intended to immerse himself in a noble contemplative tradition that rejected the niggling rules and lumbering institutions of conventional religions. When Jim arrived at the monastery, he was astounded to find everything that he disliked about religion – rigid authority structures, magical thinking, hollow ritualism, androcentrism, and petty micropolitics – firmly entrenched.

I do not offer this observation as a critique of Jim. Not at all. Each of us operates with a partial grasp of the larger context in which we find ourselves. When I was about eighteen years old, I waited for forty-five minutes at a bus stop after a soccer practice. As two busses passed me by, I became increasingly enraged as it became more and more obvious that yet again, white drivers were discriminating against poor little beige me. As the third bus passed by, I turned my head, brandished my middle finger, and swore at the driver. As I did so, I noticed out of the corner of my eye that I had been standing at a no parking sign the whole time. I burst into laughter – a fact that must have confused the gas station attendant nearby, who had been watching me quizzically. It was a humbling moment but quite useful: when

I find myself luxuriating in self-righteous indignation over a slight from a peer or friend, the memory of my minidrama with the no parking sign reminds me how often it is that strong feelings grow out of an incomplete sense of reality.

Jim survived his crisis by actively exploring the links between his personal – that is, spiritual – experiences and knowledge of Buddhism, on the one hand, and the mundane realities of organized monastic life, on the other hand. He became a superb scholar through looking carefully for the fascinating links between regional politics and economics and Buddhist philosophical and ritual lifeways. To put it another way – when he abandoned the idea that his beloved Buddha had inspired a community that was uniquely free from the irrationalities of other institutions, he could adopt what one might call a Buddhism for adults.

Magic and Adulthood

It seems fair to note that the critical orientation that is the modus operandi of scholarly life is not a major feature of yogaland. In my conversation with Jack, I suggested, "But isn't it always better for people to have more rather than less knowledge about what they're doing and saying?" As I reflect on the experiences that I have had since 2013, especially on those that I have had during the more intensive period of fieldwork over the past two years, this innocent question seems more complicated (and more naive).

Jack's response, "I just wonder if it might mess with a person's experience if they got too bogged down in the details," captures the dilemma perfectly. The subtext of my question, of course, is whether knowledge about texts, ideas, communities, practices, and rituals oriented toward religious – or for that matter, toward spiritual or mystical – elements necessarily wrecks a person's experience or even just threatens to wreck it?

I do not think that there is an easy answer to the first part of this question, yet the answer to the second part is yes, at least for me. A certain kind of knowledge does *threaten* to disenchant or radically flatten one's experience. What I have in mind is the kind of knowledge that explains the feelings, convictions, habits, institutions, and origin stories of religious insiders *in terms of other* (specifically, nondivine) forces. These kinds of explanations are the stock-in-trade of the academic study of religion. Most of us do not advance historical or sociological accounts of religion in order to ruin the feelings, convictions, and communal bonds of the people we study. But of course, most of us do assume that when a creationist hears their first rock-solid account of human evolution, they will feel at least a little, well, doubtful about the stories that they have held dear since they were a child.

I think that most of my peers also expect that when someone first learns about Durkheim's notions of *communitas* and collective effervescence – concepts that describe how people have elevated feelings of love, transcendence, and solidarity when gathered at special events – they will likely have second (or at least some complex) thoughts the next time that they experience these feelings in a church or a yoga studio. Suffice it to say that the core theories of Karl Marx, Émile Durkheim, Sigmund Freud, Max Weber, Friedrich Nietzsche, feminists, and even the sometimes shrill "new atheists" (e.g., Richard Dawkins, Christopher Hitchens, and Sam Harris) at the very least give some religious people pause – and for good reason.

There are in fact many innovative and respectable ways that religious insiders can and do reimagine their ideas, feelings, beliefs, and habits upon hearing theories or sustaining traumas that challenge previous certainties.[29] At least for me, it does not seem at all tenable to maintain one's original innocent perspective – born of one's family origins or of one's dramatic adult conversion, for example – in the face of the many truths articulated by the critics above, who promise more, rather than less, knowledge about what they are doing and saying as religious people.

Nonetheless, I am not satisfied with a definitive flat atheism that one might assume is the natural by-product of "mess[ing] with a person's experience" (to use Jack's turn of phrase). Perhaps what I am describing is just a conventional example of the quintessential modern predicament of people finding themselves somewhat ill at ease with all comprehensive solutions. Still, I continue to feel – and it is just a feeling, for better and for worse – unsure about how or why one would continue with one's practice, whether it be Christian prayer, Buddhist meditation, or postural yoga, without some reimagined sense of awe, curiosity, joy, transcendence, and sacredness; readers should imagine scare quotes around these terms.

Of course, the situation may be different for people raised in a deeply rooted ethnoreligious community; here, I am imagining Hindus, Jews,

Muslims, Sikhs, Mennonites, Anglicans, and Catholics, for example. In that case, one might feel an attachment to one's family or ethnic group. The affective and social components of such forms of religiosity are strong and may be sufficient to keep people engaged communally following the disenchantment often produced through sober critical inquiry or traumatic experiences. But for those of us who join groups as adults and who do not have any familial nostalgia for incense, culturally specific foods, gurus, or a particular asana sequence, what happens when knowledge challenges or simply contradicts one's sense of wonder? What, then, might it mean to leave, or to stay in, such a place?

Conclusion

Religion, spirituality, and secularity are never neutral things-in-themselves but always concepts that have what we might call site-specific and time-specific meanings.[30] Above, we have seen the ways that the key terms religion and spirituality are often juxtaposed: yoga is (or I am) spiritual but not religious. However, this juxtaposition itself is not a statement of fact (like "India is in Asia, not in North America") but an argument (more like "India is spiritual, whereas America is materialistic"). The spirituality-versus-religion juxtaposition that I heard many dozens of times in my research makes sense only against the backdrop of the assumption that the former is the liberating solution to the inherently conformist and backward-looking tendencies of the latter. Fair enough, but this relatively new backdrop was built very recently in and for the liberal democratic West. Elsewhere, the relationship between religion and spirituality is understood – or "constructed" – quite differently.

In chapter 5, I address this difference at length, but when defining yoga in North America as, for example, spiritual, religious, Asian, global, or commercial, one is often also saying something about yoga in South Asia. After all, the links – real and imagined – between yoga in ancient India and yoga in contemporary Miami are what make what happens in the latter space identifiable as yoga rather than stretching, as the Iyengar teacher Joanne remarked above.

But here, it is important to pay attention to the distinctive features of the Indian backdrop against which one might make some kind of claim about what yoga is and is not. In the roughly hundred years that have passed between Krishnamacharya's arrival at the Mysore Palace and today, Indian and North American societies have changed dramatically. The birth of modern India as an ostensibly secular (but majority Hindu) state unfolded between the middle of the nineteenth and the middle of the twentieth centuries. In (roughly) the second half of this period, modern postural yoga was newly consolidated in India and then was brought to and reimagined in a North American society where there was already some nascent interest in yoga and other "Oriental" traditions and techniques.[31] The roots of these plants cannot be disentangled.

The excitement that occasioned the state's emergence in 1947 was obviously quickly overshadowed by real-world political events such as Mohandas Gandhi's assassination in 1948, tensions with an also new Pakistan, and the horrific fallout associated with the mass migration of millions of people to and from India and Pakistan during the partition.

The list could be much longer, of course, but the point is that the consolidation of postural yoga in South Asia occurred during decades of turmoil and bloodshed that are almost impossible to compare with the social changes unfolding in Canada and the United States in the same period. Just as India struggled to realize its independence after centuries of resource extraction by British overlords, Canada and the United States were in periods of rapid expansion and (in the latter case) en route to becoming the preeminent global superpower.

Nonetheless, during the expansion of postural yoga in North America over roughly the past fifty years, most teachers and students have reached a kind of unspoken consensus that yoga should not be too tightly identified with Indic religions. Such a shared perspective emerged over decades and appealed to yoga enthusiasts in Canada and the United States who had begun to view religion with real and often well-earned suspicion. I suspect that the founders of modern postural yoga, such as Krishnamacharya, would not have thought of asana practice as a spiritual or secular (or post- or antireligious) activity in the ways that so many contemporary Canadians and Americans do. In fact, the early South Asian exporters of Patanjali's yoga might have thought that Western practitioners had missed the point of the practice almost entirely by focusing so much on asanas and eschewing most religionish or bhakti (theistic and devotional) features. Nevertheless, this speculation should not distract us from the broad consensus mentioned above.

Over the past hundred years, the sands of religion, spirituality, and secularity have shifted differently in North America than they have in South Asia, and one always needs to bear these differences in mind before assuming that the same concepts can be used in multiple settings. It is certainly peculiar that contemporary North American practitioners, who say that they have no interest in the religious history of yoga, make regular use of images, ideas, texts, sounds, teaching styles, and practices that are clearly derived from Hinduism, Buddhism, Tantrism, and Jainism. But ironies abound in India too: through the Ministry of Ayurveda, Yoga and Naturopathy, Unani, Siddha and Homoeopathy (AYUSH), the *Common Yoga Protocol*, and the International Day of Yoga, Patanjali's ostensibly apolitical yoga has become, as it were, yoked to the interests of Indian politicians, as Andrea Jain and others have observed.

Practitioners are never really alone on their mats. When I find some floor space in the shala, I know that I am joined by all of my biases, privileges, and habits, which in turn shape the way that I hear words such as religious and spiritual and also their synonyms (e.g., sacred) and antonyms (e.g., secular). Next to me in my shala, I find former fundamentalist Christians, people blending Sikhism and Anglicanism, New Age energy workers, and many people who are utterly indifferent to all things religious.

I have traced the reasons why the religionish dimensions of postural yoga practice are often referred to as spiritual, or even secular, when they are referred to at all, which is not often. My curiosity about exactly how we agree to use a certain set of words, gestures, and habits in studios obviously reflects my own background and training but might be of some use as I introduce other aspects of yogaland, such as superpowers. It seems to me that the most interesting conversations occur not when one tries to critique or defend a certain term but when one asks someone what they mean when they refer

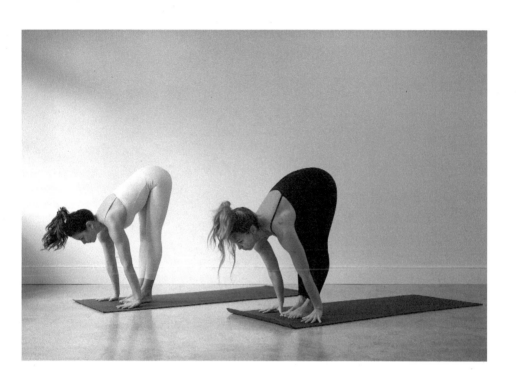

Figure 2.2
Ardha uttanasana (half forward fold pose)

to something as spiritual rather than religious. Usually, the answer amounts to a critique of how our society's dominant religious institutions and norms (especially Christianity) have hurt them or imperilled the planet and how a properly spiritual yoga practice might liberate us all. It turns out that what seems like a story about the shifting meaning of words is actually or also a story about how we respond to political as well as personal traumas.

CHAPTER THREE

The Body Settles the Score

You do not have to be good.
You do not have to walk on your knees
for a hundred miles through the desert repenting.
You only have to let the soft animal of your body
love what it loves.
Tell me about despair, yours, and I will tell you mine.
Mary Oliver[1]

I went into the field looking for evidence of the differences between postural yoga in the United States and Canada. These dissimilarities are interesting, but it became clear right away that students and teachers did not think very often about these matters on their own. What they do think about is their bodies, their practices, their communities, and their wishes to be whole.

I did not expect to meet so many wounded, soft animals, as Mary Oliver might have said. But there I was – bearing witness to story after story of trauma, brokenness, alienation, humiliation, and eventual (if often only in-complete) recovery. I do not know why these stories surprised me. After all, I did not end up on a yoga mat because I was bored one day or wanted to lose weight. I am a child of Albert Camus, Emmanuel Levinas, Elie Wiesel, and Friedrich Nietzsche, and so I am predisposed to think that life contains a great deal of, or perhaps simply amounts to, suffering.

But to have suffering as a central topographical feature of my mental map is different than to hear again and again exactly how a specific person sitting across from me on a yoga bolster was brought low by a divorce or, for that matter, the death of a child, an abortion, a stillbirth, sexual violence or manipulation, flagrant racism, a car accident, marital abuse, depression, anxiety, obsessive compulsive disorder, multiple sclerosis, scoliosis, arthritis, bullying, inherited effects of colonization, an addiction to alcohol, heroin, crack, nicotine, or cocaine, an eating disorder, cancer, abusive parenting, extreme poverty, diabetes, morbid obesity, or an attempted suicide.

This is an abridged list. Once the question of well-being arose in interviews and focus groups, the stories poured out. Whenever this happened, I heard Oliver's words in my mind: Tell me about despair, yours, and I will tell you mine.

By tacit consensus, most of us agree to act as though these stories are exceptional. Such a charade allows us to take care of mundane responsibilities, but it is nonetheless false.

In the previous chapter, I described my first "half primary" class. This was a turning point for me, and so I decided that I would keep attending those Friday evening classes. The next week, I showed up, found a place in the back row, and listened as Jack explained a deep-breathing technique that is part of many yoga traditions. In Ashtanga, practitioners are normally instructed to constrict the back of the throat somewhat and to breathe as though one were trying to fog up a mirror. Of course, doing so means that one's breathing is more audible than it would otherwise be. After explaining this approach, Jack led the Sanskrit invocation and guided us through the set sequence of asanas. I found it difficult and unnatural to constrict my throat, hold difficult postures, and use only my nose to breathe, but I could certainly feel the benefits. It drew my attention to my breath – which is to say, it drew my attention away from the citta vritti (endless whirlpool of thoughts) – and quickly began to increase the heat in my body.

Within five minutes, however, another fact crowded everything else out of my mind: there was a guy in the front row whose breathing was twice as loud as everyone else's. He was four rows in front of me, and as in the previous week, the lights were low, so I could not see him clearly. Still, I could tell both that he was in his late twenties and that he was a very strong practitioner. He had the ability to float slowly backward as he moved from uttanasana (standing forward fold pose) to chaturanga dandasana (low plank pose; see figure 3.1), for example. And then he could float his body forward from adho mukha shvanasana (downward-facing dog pose) such that his feet would leave the floor at the back of the mat and land without a sound between his hands at the front of the mat. These are skills that very few students can master. He was clearly trying to show the class, and Jack, that he was an advanced practitioner in every sense: he moved and breathed more effectively, more deeply, than everyone else. I tried not to watch him, but his breathing was extremely loud and his movements seemed to defy the laws of physics, so it was hard to focus on my own practice.

During utthita hasta padangusthasana (extended hand-to-big-toe pose; see figure 3.2), I found myself looking for the clock on the wall, wishing that the class would end so that I could stop being an audience member for this guy. An elaborate story about him developed in my mind. I could just imagine him bragging about his local, raw, vegan diet in the change room, his summers spent tree planting, his trips to India, his trust fund, and his winters spent training for a pentathlon. During shavasana (corpse pose), I had to work hard not to clench my jaw since this student's breathing actually became louder when we all stopped moving. It struck me that he was taking advantage of the last opportunity to show us how serious he was about his practice.

As I rolled up my mat, I was irritated that my mind could not settle and that this class felt so different from the same one just a week before. I imagined the conversation that I would have when I got home. "How was it?" my partner would probably ask. "It is the end of my innocence, I guess. The spell is broken," I planned to say. Perhaps it was a bit strange to rehearse this response during shavasana, but I was discouraged, and imagining this conversation gave my mind something to do.

As I trudged from the practice room to the change room, I avoided making eye contact with Jack, who had been so kind with me in the previous months, since I did not want to tell him how aggravated I was by the pretentious show-off in the front row. Instead, I walked past him and opened the curtain to the men's change-room. There, the lights were on and people

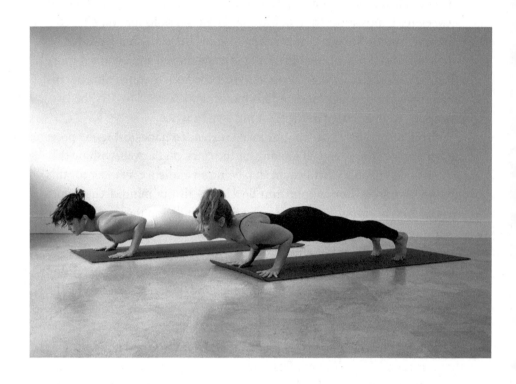

Figure 3.1
Chaturanga dandasana (low plank pose)

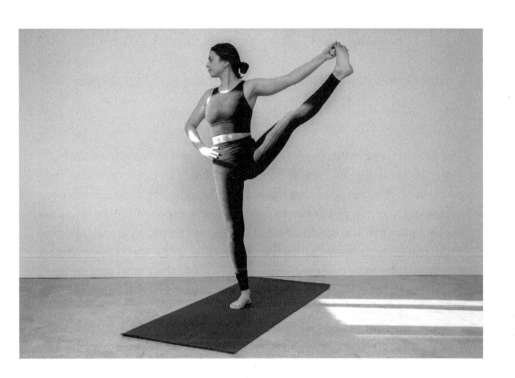

Figure 3.2
Utthita hasta padangusthasana (extended hand-to-big-toe pose)

were chatting amiably about their plans for the weekend. I was silent and grumpy as I sat down heavily on a bench to put on my socks.

"Oops. Sorry, dude," someone said as he brushed by me in the cramped change room.

I looked up. Eighteen inches in front of me was the naked torso of the heavy breather. Before I could finish saying "No problem," I saw it. He had a half-inch-thick scar running from just below his throat all the way to his belly button.

Half an hour later when I got home, my partner did ask, "So, how was it?"

"Bad news. Turns out I'm not as good a person as I had thought."

The fact that we use the word "trauma" so often and so broadly says something about another consensus that has developed in our society over the past two or three decades: that many of us struggle with deep tears in our emotional, mental, physical, or spiritual fabric. Some of the tears in the list above are medical conditions that come from within a person's genetic code, some are assaults inflicted from outside, some are random accidents, and some are the result of ideologies. All of these tears are traumas in the sense of being wounds,[2] but what really matters is what happens after the scarring incident.

The Centre for Addictions and Mental Health in Toronto offers a conventional elaboration: "Trauma is the lasting emotional response that often results from living through a distressing event."[3] Psychiatrist Judith Herman's *Trauma and Recovery: The Aftermath of Violence from Domestic Abuse to Political Terror* (1992) helped to lay the groundwork for our thinking about the links between personal and political violence, on the one hand, and maladaptive approaches to life, on the other hand, with a special interest in the ways that the trauma often occasions dissociation. In his book *The Trauma of Everyday Life* (2013), psychiatrist Mark Epstein makes the case for broadening our definition of trauma from a mental state following an unusual and dramatic *event* to a feature of every human life.[4]

Whether the source is in one's genes, a dark alley, one's own mind, or one's family, traumatic events feel overwhelming; that is their primary characteristic. Religious studies scholar Tamsin Jones observes the overlap between major religious experiences (such as conversions and epiphanies) and trauma narratives, noting that both are "unbidden" and disorienting. Fundamentally, both types of experiences challenge "the subject's ability to integrate the event into a world of meaning, to know or understand what they underwent, or to speak about it, [which] causes a kind of death of that former self." This outcome of trauma helps us to appreciate how the ruptures that I heard about almost every day during fieldwork expelled people from life as they knew it and often left them ready for something radically new.[5]

But consider the extravagant imagery here: rupture, death, tear, unbidden, disorienting, distress, violence, assault, dissociate, inflict, upheaval, crisis. In the face of the wounds sustained by the people I met, the mind reaches for metaphors to convey experiences that seem impossible to capture, precisely because it is the nature of trauma to exceed one's capacity to communicate. The heavy breather's dramatic scar was a trauma in the sense of a wound, but usually when we use the term, we connote the "lasting emotional response" that follows the injury – not the absent or abusive parents but their impact; not the sexual humiliation but its impact.[6]

For this book, I used a powerful software system (NVivo) to manage thousands of pages of verbatim transcripts and fieldnotes. I could produce a table tracking whenever the words trauma and associated words or phrases (e.g., assault, scar, and overwhelming abuse) were used, by whom (i.e., young, old, woman, man, affluent, educated, and so on), and how long this part of the conversation lasted. However, such an illustration would tell us only what is already quite clear, namely that these stories were part of almost every conversation.

They were so ubiquitous that at the end of discussions in which the theme did not arise, as the research assistant and I were packing up and putting on our shoes, I would casually observe how often we heard harrowing stories. Almost always, my casual observation would initiate a new conversation in which the student or teacher would say something like, "Oh! I didn't really realize you were interested in *that*!" – after which they would tell us in some detail about how yoga had helped them to recover from serious physical or psychological ruptures.

It is common to think of the body as an essentially personal – and private – possession or site of experience. After all, your left knee, lower back, liver, genitals, and brain are nothing if not incontrovertibly *yours*; you determine whether they are replaced, tattooed, pierced, drugged, caressed, or donated. What happens to, and through, these parts of your body is entirely your business.

Except, that is not entirely true, is it? Consider some of the more obvious times when someone else has control: when you are in a coma, when you are a thirteen-year-old Jehovah's Witness refusing a blood transfusion, when you receive a payment for gestating someone else's fertilized egg, when you want to terminate your pregnancy but live in one of the many US states where abortion is illegal, when you want to marry two consenting adults, when you ask health care providers to help you end your life, when you sunbathe naked in New York's Central Park, or when you are penalized by your supervisor for refusing vaccines that public health officials deem crucial.

These cases remind us that our bodies are of great interest to many other people, many of whom wield the power of the state. Although our bodies are ultra-private, they are also broadly political. We vulnerable, finite, suffering soft animals live within and are conditioned by national borders, legal regimes, municipal regulations, and – most ambiguously – community standards. To understand postural yoga in North America, we need to think through what it means in these societies for bodies that are both public and private to be in yoga spaces that are both in the world and anti-world.

During interviews, focus groups, and my time in many spaces in yogaland before and after my official fieldwork period, two names came up more than any others: Bessel van der Kolk (b. 1943), a Dutch-born American psychiatrist; and Gabor Maté (b. 1944), a Hungarian-born Canadian family physician and addictions specialist. People referred to them directly or to their famous books – van der Kolk's *The Body Keeps the Score: Brain, Mind, and Body in the Healing of Trauma* (2014) and (less often) Maté's *In the Realm of Hungry Ghosts: Close Encounters with Addiction* (2008) or his *The Myth of Normal: Trauma, Healing, and Illness in a Toxic Culture* (2022). Sometimes the people we met would refer to trauma theory and theorists without naming them – in which case, I would sometimes ask the yoga students or teachers whom they had in mind, and almost always people would name van der Kolk or Maté.[7]

It is hard to overstate the influence of these two charismatic physicians whose medical insights and personal experiences are central to how people sustain and overcome their injuries and addictions and to how (in some cases) they are able to lead better lives. Both physicians and their books have had major impacts within the wellness world but also in the broader public conversation about trauma and its effects on the body. Although they readily speak in medical terms – making reference to the limbic system, serotonin, neuroreceptors, and adverse childhood events, as well as to the social factors that lead to illness and addiction – they do so in a manner that appeals to yogis, acupuncturists, reiki masters, herbalists, Wiccans, chaplains, and addictions counsellors. Indeed, their claims have become taken-for-granted aspects of yogaland. The appeal of these texts and metaphors to North American yogis is evident in a comment made by Eva, a teacher in Los Angeles:

Right. *The Body Keeps the Score.* Yep. It's an incredible book and it's absolutely accurate on every level. And when you go through any sort of trauma in your life, from my experience, your body holds onto that. Whether it's in your back, in your shoulders, in your stomach, in your hips, whatever it is. And you hold onto those emotions, and so moving your body and opening up and breathing allows you to kind of release some of that tension that your body holds onto.[8]

Another woman we met in Toronto underlined the ways that this line of thinking has been absorbed into the broader yoga scene:

I would say that … negative emotions, trauma, it gets stored in the body. *We know that.* And so the first thing I would say with somebody who's traumatized is you need to, like, deal with the, with the body first. Because if your body is heavy and in pain, it really is very hard to move to feeling love, [not to mention] feeling cared about or caring about your neighbour, because you are in pain yourself.

On the webpage associated with *The Body Keeps the Score*, one finds endorsements from esteemed psychiatrists and psychologists as well as from self-help luminaries, including Jack Kornfield (celebrated Buddhist practitioner), Stephen Cope (founder of the Kripalu Yoga Institute, who is mentioned in this book's introduction), and Jon Kabat-Zinn (famous for his work on mindfulness).[9] A physician I know observed that the title captures the argument of the book so well that many people feel that they have read the book without ever having picked it up.

These authors and texts offer a new approach to trauma that has appealed to millions of people in the larger culture. Although van der Kolk, Maté, and other contributors to the conversation, such as Epstein and Herman, have different backgrounds, interests, and styles, it is worthwhile to think of these books and authors as an amalgam since the yoga teachers and students we interviewed often invoked them together and credited them with the same core insights. In short, it is by now received wisdom in yogaland and well beyond – even among people who have never read the book of the same name or heard the name of its author – that the body keeps the score.

These writers argue that almost all of us have borne such traumatic damages and that most of us have survived through dissociation, in which the victim hives off some aspect of their minds. Consequently, the key features of the trauma – what its impacts have been, what it felt like, why or even where it happened, who is responsible, how one might pursue justice or reconciliation – are not integrated into the larger story of one's life. Although the trauma remains in some sense opaque to its victim, it expresses itself in often devastating mental and physical maladies (e.g., depression, anxiety, addiction, fibromyalgia, suicidality, and hypertension), as well as in deeply maladaptive approaches to other people (e.g., rage, submissiveness, and infidelity).

Advances in tools and methods such as sleep studies, functional magnetic resonance imaging, heart rate variability monitors, blood pressure monitoring, and structured psychological interviews mean that we understand better than ever before the effect of trauma on a person's limbic system and a vast array of connected bodily systems such as the skin, gastrointestinal system, and cardiovascular system. Nonetheless, we are still in the early phases of our comprehension of these injuries, and as van der Kolk points out, there has been resistance from some – fewer and fewer, it appears – of his medical peers to coming to terms with trauma as a specific sort of injury with a specific sort of impact.

The demonstrable limitations of conventional forms of treatment have also helped us to appreciate the way that social factors such as poverty, racism, dysfunctional families, and limited access to education and healthy food generate and exacerbate illness. Over the past few decades, scientists and clinicians have begun to understand better why trauma seems somewhat resistant both to major pharmaceutical options (e.g., selective serotonin reuptake inhibitors, or SSRIs, such as Prozac) and to the "talking cure," in which the traumatic event is the focus of direct discussion and debate.

Since the event haunts our limbic system and interferes with our perception of the world by skewing our capacity to understand what is and is not a threat, one needs to approach it indirectly, doing so through the body. As van der Kolk contends:

> Being traumatized means continuing to organize your life as if the trauma were still going on – unchanged and immutable – as every new encounter or event is contaminated by the past. After trauma, the world is experienced with a different nervous system. The survivor's energy now becomes focused on suppressing inner chaos, at the expense of spontaneous involvement in their life … These attempts to maintain control over unbearable physiological reactions can result in a whole range of physical symptoms … This explains why it is critical for trauma treatment to engage the entire organism, body, mind, and brain.[10]

Mounting evidence of the ubiquity of trauma has bolstered alternative health regimes such as yoga, mindfulness, acupuncture, and reiki that promise to address suffering in a way that conventional biomedicine does not. There are now hundreds of graduate degrees, certificates, workshops, textbooks, videos, seminars, and protocols dedicated to "trauma-informed" and "trauma-sensitive" therapy, pedagogy, policing, business administration, coaching, public administration, social services, and health care. Of course, there is significant heterogeneity among these offerings, materials, and teachers, but there is a broad tendency to eschew directive, domineering interventions; so, for example, a trauma-informed yoga teacher would not demand or impose specific asanas but would invite and encourage students to try them and would also present alternatives.[11]

Yoga students and teachers sometimes say "the body keeps the score" by way of an explanation of why their headaches, joint problems, anxiety, and depression did not respond well to conventional therapeutic interventions such as physiotherapy, medication, talk therapy, or surgery. According to a story told often enough that it became a trope in this project, the chief problem of these common therapies is their atomistic approach to the body and its illnesses. Books and workshops on trauma-informed teaching and healing modalities help students and teachers to understand that they are not getting better largely because conventional interventions do not treat the person as a whole and do not adequately address either the roots of trauma or where the trauma is stored.

So people turn elsewhere – to their friends, the Internet, yoga studios, and their own intuition. There, they learn that conventional approaches to wellness and illness are misguided and inadequately attentive to the wisdom of the patient and their body. As a reflection of the ways that the body both keeps the score and tells a story, practitioners would often say, "My body was telling me something," when they spoke about how yoga helped them to recover from an illness that conventional modalities could not cure.

Readers will be familiar with the basic principle that physical symptoms (e.g., hives) often reflect psychological states (e.g., anxiety). Van der Kolk goes beyond this psychosomatic theory and focuses on traumatic events as the origins of both mental states and physical symptoms. Martha, a hot yoga teacher in Indiana, reflected on the ways that many of us are disconnected from our bodies: "There are a lot of people who are, you know, [they] experience a lot of trauma in their bodies. Like sometimes you give them a cue, and you have to give them the same cue three or four times before they can translate it into what you're asking them to do with their bodies."

Martha's story reflected my own experience of learning about body-mind disconnection and the challenges of proprioception.[12] I once watched a teacher use many variations of the same cue – "turn your back foot out to the left" – with a Japanese student. Eventually, the teacher had to use her hand to move the student's foot three inches to the left. In my new-student hubris, I thought that I should take the teacher aside to explain that Kenji was clearly having a hard time understanding her English instructions.

My teacher was patient with me yet matter-of-fact in her response. "I doubt it. He has been living and working here for seven years, and he certainly knows what 'foot,' 'left,' 'move,' and 'your' mean. He just doesn't have a very good connection between his mind and his body, so it takes him a really long time to connect what I am saying with what his body can do."

A senior vinyasa teacher in British Columbia, Katrine, referred to her own trauma but noted, "Nobody was talking about trauma [in the late 1990s]. And I also hadn't really talked to that many people about my experience. And so, you know, I wasn't sleeping, and [I was] grinding my teeth at night, and, uh, I started just kind of living in the yoga studio … The type of yoga that I was doing, it wasn't particularly spiritual, but we were moving our bodies, and … I realized in one particular class when we were in shavasana that it was the first time I had any sense of relaxation for a year."

The asana teachers and students I met described many types of traumas. Whether they use "evidence-based" biomedicine or complementary health practices to cope with them, they all spoke of the ways that their injuries clung to their bodies. To echo something from chapter 1, those bodies *do not live nowhere*, so it would be worthwhile to place these bodies within a broader context.

The Yoga Body on the Map

Earlier, I outlined the ways that yoga studios are liminal anti-worlds inasmuch as they (at least on the surface) provide an oasis from the loud, fast, and dirty aspects of the world outside the studio. Of course, as with other popular escapes – all-inclusive spas, Disneyland, most weddings, and the Muslim pilgrimage (hajj), for example – the regular world, with its capitalism, patriarchy, and so forth, is still present to a large degree. Nonetheless, the distinction between world and anti-world is meaningful and palpable. For this reason, practitioners regularly reported having had powerful and sometimes life-changing experiences in these spaces that they might not have been able to have elsewhere. If we are to understand what makes studios so appealing for traumatized students, we need to ask what makes the surrounding society traumatogenic.[13]

A Patchwork of Precarities

During and in the years just prior to this study, Canadians and Americans have been mired in their respective existential crises. Some are rather state-specific, and others are much broader. As I consider what I heard during fieldwork and in conversations over the past decade in yogaland, it seems to me that we can organize these concerns from (roughly) the global to the local. Below I offer a list of these sources of distress, with a more thorough explication provided of those issues that were of greater concern to the people we met.

Climate Change

Canadians and Americans have seen "atmospheric rivers" on the West Coast, landslides, floods, fires, droughts, and other extreme weather events. Although there is some evidence that policy makers and consumers are beginning to take both notice and action, some of us understandably worry that the response will be too little and come too late. Study after study, as well as the front-line clinical experience of mental-health workers and teachers in public education, confirm the ubiquity and severity of climate grief, climate despair, and eco-anxiety.

These conditions are not just diagnosable but also now endemic, with consequences that mirror the ways that van der Kolk frames trauma.[14] As Charlie Hertzog Young writes, "It's hard to imagine what could be more traumatic than near-death experiences, the decimation of your community, home and livelihood, let alone the loss of loved ones, forced migration, or being caught in the crossfire of conflict. Climate breakdown is driving an uptick in all of these."[15] The American Psychiatric Association echoes these impressions: "The mental health consequences of events linked to a changing global climate include mild stress and distress, high-risk coping behavior such as increased alcohol use and, occasionally, mental disorders such as depression, anxiety and post-traumatic stress."[16]

I doubt that I need to provide a long litany of the devastation – real and impending – associated with climate change. I raise this matter because the precarity of our climate is surely both a geotechnical problem and a political dilemma, with prolonged exposure to dark forecasts about the collapse of the world as we know it being potentially not just stressful but also traumatic, as many teachers and students observed.

The Growth of Populism

In the past decade, we have witnessed a troubling growth not just in extreme political rhetoric (usually, yet not always, from the right wing) but also in policies, leaders, and priorities designed to capitalize on extreme orientations. In the United States in particular the political system has become deeply polarized and has focused on dramatic issues associated with the so-called culture wars (e.g., debates in the United States regarding whether elementary school books should promote "critical race theory"). The resulting gridlock is not quite as dire in Canada as it is in the United States, but American economic and political might means that many people outside of that society share in the strife created mainly within it.

Colonial Legacies

Many North Americans are reckoning with the impact of our colonial histories. In Canada, the 2015 report of the Truth and Reconciliation Commission of Canada was the culmination of the Supreme Court's mandated assessment of the legacy of Indigenous residential schools. The eight-year cross-country process was governed by Indigenous leaders and involved regular news coverage, political engagement, and public hearings with Indigenous groups, survivors, and their kin, as well as with representatives of the Christian denominations that had managed the schools. The often-graphic hearings, debates, healing circles, apologies, and settlements unfolded in real time and often in public.

This process, which dovetails with the work of van der Kolk and Maté, led to a heightened awareness of the "intergenerational trauma" that shows up in the minds and bodies of Indigenous people today. I mention the process of truth and reconciliation to illustrate a main feature of the political zeitgeist of Canada for the past fifteen years, one that both overlaps with the rise of yoga practice in Canada and has occasioned some national soul-searching.

Whereas US society has yet to address its treatment of Indigenous people in a comprehensive manner on par with the work of the Truth and Reconciliation Commission, one could say that the Black Lives Matter movement – which began in 2012 and vastly expanded after the 2020 police killing of George Floyd – represented an expression of rage and resistance against a society that often stifles African American citizens and communities. Clearly, Black Lives Matter builds on larger civil rights movements in the United States, part of the unfinished labour of pioneers such as Martin Luther King Jr. This is not the place to address this movement or Canada's commission in depth, but it is worth considering both as reflections of North America's traumatogenic colonial project.

The Neoliberal Turn

Margaret Thatcher, Ronald Reagan, Brian Mulroney, and many others who followed them weakened the social safety net that had been built over the decades following the Second World War. The "Washington Consensus"[17] captures the policies and programs advocated by the confident common-sense neoliberalism that emerged in the 1980s. That "people should pick themselves up by their bootstraps" was a conviction often expressed in the years when we witnessed the attenuation of protections offered to workers, the poor, and the environment. This neoliberal turn unfolded at the same time as the expansion of those varieties of globalization that, among other things, unfettered corporations.[18] As with the Enlightenment, this new social order was expected (by those who championed it) to increase wealth, individual freedoms, women's latitude, and democracy, but without the cradle-to-grave protection of the "nanny state" (to use a dismissive term common among neoliberals in these decades), the individual would be increasingly on his or her own.[19]

Other commentators are better able to outline the shortcomings of this ideological orientation.[20] However, it is worth noting that the bootstrap metaphor was originally understood to underline the impossibility of some task. In truth, one is born into and is, for better or worse, dependent on a web of relationships, from intimate relations with one's friends and family to less familiar affiliations with one's neighbours, teachers, employers, and the government officials and ministries that build and maintain roads, hospitals, and water treatment facilities.

One might not feel well supported by one's family and society, but no one pulls themselves up by their bootstraps, or fails to do so, on their own. The bootstrap metaphor now rather flatly refers to people whose grit and determination allow them to overcome formidable obstacles. The semantic flattening of this metaphor is a perfect, if also ironic, illustration of the normalization and invisibilization of neoliberalism as an ideology that does what all ideologies do, namely narrow one's vision.

The problem is not just what trauma does to an individual's body and mind but also the ways that injury takes the individual out of their society, leaving them in a state of anomie, normless, and disconnected from community. In this state, we are vulnerable to market forces that pit us against one another. Speaking to the dire consequences of anomie (and echoing the key insights of Maté), Scottish journalist Johann Hari contends, "The opposite of addiction is not sobriety – it's human connection."[21]

A clear indication of the neoliberal turn is the tendency to see oneself as a brand that needs to be curated and marketed. This sensibility is deeply embedded in the Canadian and American yoga scenes, with slick websites featuring ultra-capable, beautifully sculpted, young, and most often white female bodies.[22] Studio owners are further pressured by the fact that everyone is competing for the same students and teachers, with virtually no labour protections for staff and usually very thin profit margins.[23] Innumerable people I have met – in this project and in my time in yogaland – distrust the market, with its values of individualism, hedonism, materialism, and competition, yet all recognize that in order to survive, they are trapped by the aesthetic and economic rules of the game.

Health Care Anxieties

The economic precarity occasioned by neoliberalism seemed to affect everyone we met in similar ways. However, in the United States, practitioners had the additional and significant burden of health care to worry about. For me, one of the most perplexing features of our US fieldwork was hearing story after story of financial precarity or ruin caused by inadequate or expensive health care. American readers will not be surprised by most of these stories. Here is some of what we heard:

- One teacher spoke of the ways that long-married couples would divorce and shift assets to the healthy partner in order to enable the ailing partner to have access to Medicare services.
- A younger participant spoke of not getting married because it would mean that she would need to leave Medicaid, which would add costs to her husband's private insurance.
- A senior yoga teacher spoke of his quite good private coverage, which nonetheless left him worried about whether "a bill for $65,000 will come in the mail" weeks or months after he had left the hospital.[24]
- A graduate student on a comprehensive state health plan for low-income people spoke about how her (basic) prescriptions are not accepted by almost any pharmacy within easy driving distance of her home.
- One young teacher, despite having health insurance, spoke about how the direct costs of treatment for her (common) cancer had not only required her to mount a GoFundMe campaign but had also required her father to make negotiating with insurance providers his full-time job during her year-long treatment.
- Several spoke of how they would accept or remain in jobs for years longer than they would prefer just to ensure that they had access to care since health care arrangements are dependent on one's employer.[25]
- One military veteran with excellent coverage, after cutting her knee badly while hiking, drove herself to the nearest hospital for stitches and later received a bill for $8,000, much of which her own plan would not cover.
- Several participants who believed that they had good health plans spoke about how very few physicians would accept the coverage provided by the company through which they were insured.
- Curtis, a robustly healthy yoga teacher, spoke of moving from Hawaii to the Midwest strictly to get access to his partner's superior health care plan.
- A very established teacher in California who pays $600 each month for her plan and whose $7,000 deductible does not free her from

additional expenses spoke of having received an additional $25,000 bill for a one-day visit to the hospital to receive an IV drip and basic tests, treatment that did not include surgery, a diagnosis, or a cure.

This is an abridged list.[26]

I am certainly not suggesting that Canada's health care system is the pinnacle of efficiency or that it is universally loved. Throughout Canada, there are (controversial) experiments with two-tiered coverage, there is a patchwork quilt of approaches to the private delivery of nonurgent procedures, there is a severe shortage of physicians and nurses, and there is a wide variety of arrangements in the provinces regarding which medications are covered. However, as we found in our survey, Canadians who complain about the "single-payer" publicly funded system, called Medicare, generally complain about their problems with timely access to the system rather than about its ethics or economics.

What this difference between the two systems means is that the kind of health-care-based precarity that clearly distresses American yoga practitioners generally does not concern Canadians. Everyone worries, of course, about themselves or their loved ones becoming ill. Nonetheless, the direct cost of medical care can easily bankrupt Americans, whereas that is almost never a problem faced by Canadians.[27] These kinds of stories help to explain why in our survey we found that just 3 per cent of Americans thought that the US emphasis on private health care was good, whereas 69 per cent of Canadians felt the same way about their society's emphasis on public health care.

As one senior New York teacher put it, "A lot of us that are doing yoga day in and day out, we do view it as some sort of preventative something. You know, I would like to stay away from the hospital as much as possible, not only for my own health but just because I don't want all the freaking [financial] surprises ... [Practitioners] don't want to be bankrupt and be in debt the rest of our lives."

Sexual Misconduct

In chapter 5, I discuss controversies within the yoga world with regard to sexual abuse, appropriate boundaries between teachers and students, and gender and sexual diversities. For now, I can note that yoga's #MeToo movement might have been framed as a way to identify transgressions of (mostly) powerful men against (mostly) women, but it obviously created a broad conversation within many societies about systemic injustices faced by women. The disorientation and pain that came into view with these scandals forced many students and teachers, over 80 per cent of them women, to decide whether in fact yogaland was safer than – or exactly as unsafe as – the rest of their society. Their answers led to a reckoning in some communities. The Anusara system, for example, essentially vanished when complaints surfaced against its leader; as well, in the Ashtanga system, the prominence of the late Pattabhi Jois was diminished significantly.

In addition, American women in our study noted the ways that their sense of precarity was accentuated in the spring of 2021 when the US Supreme Court overturned the landmark *Roe v. Wade* decision, threatening the reproductive freedom of millions of their peers in states where abortion was consequently made illegal. Many Canadians felt solidarity with American women deeply distressed by the US Supreme Court's decision,[28] but these Canadians were at least consoled by the fact that the anti-choice movement in Canada is not a significant political or juridical force.[29]

COVID-19

Teachers and students all reflected on the profound impact of the COVID-19 pandemic on their minds, bodies, communities, studios, families, finances, and friends. The tone of the stories and the memories shared seemed somewhat darker in the United States than in Canada, likely because the death rate was more than 2.5 times higher and because vaccine hesitancy was far more politically aligned in the former society.[30]

Some enterprising teachers took advantage of the pandemic to expand their online businesses, not just offering more asana options to more students through the sudden popularity of on-line platforms but also adding to these offerings a wide array of complementary services such as muscle testing, tarot readings, teacher training, and counselling. However, even these enterprising teachers – few in number but notable nonetheless – all observed the devastation that COVID-19 rained upon the yoga world. In Los Angeles, for example, YogaWorks, one of the largest and most influential yoga franchises in North America, with fifty studios at its peak, closed the last of its studios due to COVID-19 just weeks before I visited the city for fieldwork in November 2022. Ahimsa Yoga, one of the larger studios we visited in Toronto, closed just weeks after we had visited, and many other studio owners or managers spoke openly about their fear that the community that they had built over a decade or two of hard (and not very well-remunerated) work could become unsustainable within the next few years if the pre-pandemic conditions did not return.

Several other teachers had shifted from teaching fifteen classes a week at one or two studios to teaching three or four classes at three or four studios. Some previously devoted in-person students continued to practise as much and in some cases more than they had before the pandemic, but they took a range of classes at their preferred in-person studio as well as often free online classes offered by "yogalebrities" such as Adriene Mishler, Jessamyn Stanley, and Kino MacGregor.[31] A few students I met in 2022 were still nervous about returning to studios, even those that had instituted health plans that met or exceeded those required by the local public health authorities.

Teachers felt that roughly the same number of people were practising as before the pandemic but were just doing so in different contexts and often at home, with the future of large studios being uncertain, especially those offering just one brand or denomination of yoga. It is still too early to know how COVID-19 changed the yoga world, although my impression is that the alterations were profound. It is hard to determine whether these changes were on balance good for teachers and students. It is at least possible that the pandemic inspired innovative ways of delivering asana instruction and cultivating community. Nonetheless, it was not surprising that nearly all practitioners spoke of the pandemic as a deeply disorienting and stressful time in their practice and personal lives.

The Economics of Yoga

About half of the teachers we interviewed worked exclusively as yoga teachers. The other half had several "side hustles" or full-time jobs as waiters, art teachers, physiotherapists, university professors, lawyers, models, and so forth. To sustain themselves economically, those for whom yoga was their main occupation often needed to work at several studios across the city or to take on numerous "privates," which is to say one-on-one teaching gigs, often in the homes of students. Almost all of the teachers we spoke with loved teaching and practising yoga but found it to be physically taxing and quite poorly paid and unreliable work.

The Body Settles the Score

Now that we have reflected on those aspects of Canadian and American societies that might produce distress, let us return to the body.

Above, I outlined how teachers and students – and others I have engaged with during my years in yogaland – appreciated both the way that van der Kolk and others have highlighted shortcomings in the dominant biomedical model and the way that they have focused on the body as the proverbial scorekeeper of our traumas. Risha, a teacher of South Asian heritage in Canada, observed that yoga "was a lot about coming back into my body because of childhood trauma and abuse. I just dissociated. And that's ... why yoga was enticing. It was not so much about [mastering] the postural stuff but being present [in my body]."

Julie, a senior US student who had struggled with obesity and other serious health and addictions issues, reflected during a focus group discussion,

Whenever I was really suffering through something, I would always turn to yoga. I think for me, what I, I was experiencing, like for instance, I was going through a horrible breakup, and I was in a horrible mental state, you know, and I would get on my mat, and it would, it would let all those voices in my head kind of just settle down, right? It's [a fact] that that mental, that ability to just be in my body, just be in that present moment during that practice gave me this sense of freedom that allowed me to just, like, release a lot. And maybe it is the physical movement, I don't know, but there's something about it that was allowing this kind of release of these pent-up emotions ... and it was literally the only place that I could let that go.

It seems *viscerally* – that is, in our *guts* – true to say that the body might keep a record of "the trauma of everyday life":[32] divorce, bankruptcy, assault,

106

racism, debilitating anxieties about environmental collapse, or wounds inflicted (in Canada) by church and state through Indigenous residential schools or (in the United States) by state and society during civil rights struggles. This corporeal scorecard is kept or evident in the compromised limbic system but also elsewhere throughout the body and becomes more obvious as we struggle to heal as we age. The idea that the body is the repository of our (and perhaps our ancestors') past struggles also makes sense given the intimate connections between our thoughts, emotions, and bodies, connections that are mediated by our gut biomes and by epigenetic triggers (i.e., external influences and personal choices) that interact with our genetic predispositions.[33] A key insight binding much of trauma theory together is that to survive the traumatogenic event, the mind may dissociate. That is another lesson from abuse survivors, as Risha noted above.[34]

However, there is another side to this story. Many practitioners certainly appreciate postural yoga as a means to become aware of a wide range of traumas – produced by personal wounds and by the precarities sketched above – that have taken up residence in, and are tormenting, their minds and bodies.[35] Throughout this project, people talked again and again about how the body keeps the score but also – although without quite using this word – the way that it can *settle* the score. By that I mean, the body is not only the storehouse of suffering but is also the vehicle for healing.

Echoing this insight, religious studies scholar Tamsin Jones notes,

In order to survive one must do more than talk; one must act and move, kneel, sing, eat, dance, fight, stretch, breathe. Any recovery of the self must take seriously that it is not just an idea and not just a voice floating in space; it is a body that must be resurrected, in order to be restored to life. These bodily therapies can be both defensive (self-defense classes, pushing back on a therapist) and creative (dance, yoga). In both cases, however, is contained the insight that, if it is in the body that a trauma is locked, then so too it must be in the body that it is accessed and healed.[36]

Bessel van der Kolk's *The Body Keeps the Score* includes a chapter on yoga as a response to trauma, but in my view, it is the weakest chapter in an otherwise excellent book. That is not the author's fault, really. Van der Kolk conscientiously acknowledges that it is difficult for physicians or scientists to speak confidently about the benefits of a postural yoga practice for trauma victims (that is, for most people). In his 2014 book, he admitted that scientific research on the effectiveness of yoga was underdeveloped, and it seems to me that this observation is still true a decade later.[37]

Nonetheless, he lays out the most common physical, emotional, and social benefits of postural yoga. First, through the breath work that is often integrated into asana practice, practitioners gain access to the (calming) parasympathetic nervous system. Second, through the adjustments associated with many styles, people become more at ease with others seeing and sometimes touching their bodies. Third, by following cues and maintaining balance, they improve their proprioception.[38] Fourth, by directing their attention to the fluctuations of their minds as well as their internal organs, they improve their interoception.[39] Fifth, by joining communities, they diminish anomie and alienation. Finally, by engaging with the need to focus on the physical and mental efforts occurring in the present moment, they can free themselves (even if temporarily) from the endless loop of trauma-related memories.

Based on conversations with practitioners and on my own time in yogaland, I can add a seventh way in which yoga may settle the score. By offering students the experience of mastering asanas that initially seemed to be physically impossible, communities create opportunities for practitioners to reconsider other self-limiting assumptions: that they could never pursue higher education, that they could never quiet their mind, or that their birth is polluted by original sin. Instead of being unalterable facts, perhaps these assumptions, as Doris Lessing might put it, can come to be seen as "prisons they choose to live inside."[40]

The complex philosophical rationale for yoga – not just asanas but other forms as well – has been the focus of a massive contemporary scholarship and has clearly interested some people in South Asia and elsewhere.[41] The level of intellectual sophistication required to read complex yoga texts, which historically would not have been in wide circulation among ordinary householders, was limited to a very elite subculture of almost entirely male Brahmins. There is nothing especially controversial about this observation – which was also true of the Bible for most of Christian history – but it is a reminder that outside of the din of the monastery, and aside from the thrill of scholarly seminars, the vast majority of asana practitioners are not, and probably never have been, troubled by (or even aware of) the subtleties of textual or philosophical argumentation.[42] As a result, it is not surprising that ideas and schools of thought that academics treat as distinct are in the real world mixed up in the minds and communities of practitioners.

Case in point: the people I met live in a world that is simultaneously dualistic and nondualistic. Students and teachers engaged in conversations about yoga philosophy – whether these exchanges occurred in the teacher-training program that I took or in interviews and workshops – would sometimes mention the importance of Patanjali's distinction between prakriti (material nature) and purusha (consciousness).[43] In the next breath, the same people would refer to the underlying unity of the material and immaterial and to the universe as a totality, sometimes with a nod in the direction of quantum physics, although the allusions were not very elaborate. Such a unity is supposed to become evident to people as they advance in their practice, or so the story usually goes. Indeed, it was common to hear people in studios, workshops, or interviews define the word yoga itself as union, often extrapolated as union between the individual's atman (higher self) and Brahman (ultimate reality), between mind and body, between mind, body, and spirit, between all people, between all sentient beings, or between prakriti and purusha.[44]

When practising, thinking, and teaching about yoga, I also combine all of these registers – all of these interpretations, glosses, and metaphors – into a kind of philosophical masala, or mixture of Indian spices. If someone insisted, I could probably list the distinct symbolic or ritualistic ingredients, but it would otherwise never occur to me to do so, and in the case of yoga, the chance that a student would ask anything beyond the most basic question is fairly low. The point is just that the real or apparent dichotomy between our bodies and our minds (or matter and spirit) – which is a central problem for many philosophical and theological systems, including yoga as a formal school of Indian philosophy – is not exactly a nonproblem for ordinary practitioners. It is rather the case that the problem is worked out or accommodated in ways that scholars often overlook.

It seems to me that this general scenario is indicative of other religious or spiritual traditions too. The notions of the Trinity and transubstantiation are central elements of most Christian theological systems. Moreover, thanks to an elite cadre of theologians, in roughly the past 2,000 years, innumerable theological texts and traditions have emerged to champion various justifications or explanations of these ideas. There is something at least deeply mysterious about the idea that God is both one and three and about the idea that bread and wine can become the actual body and blood of a divine incarnation. Yet, for the past several centuries, the rationales that have grown up around these central concepts have not led to a lot of open debates, hand-wringing, or big schisms for regular churchgoers. Instead, those who still attend do so for other reasons, perhaps despite these intellectually challenging notions.

After spending so much time talking with North American yogis about what animates them, what they appreciate about Indic worldviews, and what they are fixing through yoga, I sense no great urgency to resolve the problems through systematic philosophy or theology. Instead, through a yoga practice, the real suffering – whether its source is physical trauma or existential crises – can be suspended just long enough to allow people to tap into what we might call their bodily or corporealized intelligence.

In postural yoga spaces, people seek relief and ideally release from travails as profound as post-traumatic stress disorder and panic attacks or as relatively light as post-menopausal weight gain. It seemed clear from our conversations – and truth be told, from my own practice – that this solace and liberation from suffering might be ineffable; that is, literally, it might be impossible to articulate. Regardless of how partial and unsystematic one's understanding of Indian philosophy might be, the once restive body can become the site and tool par excellence for knowing and healing. The *Bhagavad Gita*, the *Yoga Sutras*, and other sources of yoga philosophy certainly articulate comprehensive perspectives on the mind, body, and surrounding world, but more than anything, it is the body that settles the score.

Here, a brief return to my own story might be of some use. I mentioned that I decided to try postural yoga after receiving the depressing news that I had a bad case of osteoarthritis. Not life-threatening but certainly life-changing. My body knew the score: the bones that met in my knees had small cracks.

Of course, some of this is genetic; my mother has arthritis but, even in her mid-eighties, nothing debilitating. I was probably going to experience osteoarthritis in the future, but it had arrived two decades earlier than anticipated.

In my case, what doctors would call "the precipitating event" is suspended in my mind with what I feel (probably incorrectly) is perfect clarity. It was a cold, dark night in March 2013, and I was coaching my eleven-year-old son's soccer team at a practice. Two large self-assured boys had treated him quite unfairly in a drill I had been overseeing. I watched them cheat as if in slow motion. I tried to correct them with humour and then with firmness, but the boys asserted themselves against my son and my coaching.

In an instant, I was no longer just on that field in Victoria but also back in Winnipeg with my own childhood bullies – who were not very precise with their racism – hurling the N-word at me, my sisters, and my father. My heart raced, my chest constricted, my adrenal glands gushed.

The Victoria boys had no idea that they were actors in a drama unfolding in my limbic system. Clearly, I did not really understand what was happening either. Instead of seeing that the boys were briefly drunk on adolescent strength and freedom, all I could see was the brutal white privilege that had left a stain in my life and had permanently scarred my older sisters. Now – my overwrought mind was certain – it was coming for my son.

The head coach was not with us that evening. With no adult eyes around to squint at me in puzzlement, I gathered the team. The two bullies were lovely boys and, I am sure, are fine young men now, but as a dyad in this environment, they were not their best selves, so to speak. Both were preternaturally gifted athletes, tall, fast, and strong, but I was still fairly fit for a forty-five-year-old. I told the team that we would spend the next fifteen minutes doing a series of short- and middle-distance sprints. Everyone groaned except the bullies, who already knew they could run much faster than everyone else.

Lost in my miasma of juvenile memory, I decided to join these drills and to win them, hoping to deflate these boys a little, to undo in some way the (minor) damage that they had done to my son, and to strike a blow against the millions of bullies throughout human history who had inflicted pain just because they could. (Clearly, my imagination had slipped free of its moorings at this point.)

And so I did that.

Immediately afterward, the boys seemed duly chastened, and the rest of the practice proceeded as usual. The next day, my joints and muscles were sore, and initially I reasoned that this was a small price to pay to correct what had happened that night on the field. However, the discomfort clung to me for months. My muscles eventually stopped aching, but my joints felt swollen and bruised. The pain was relentless. I tried ice, rest, activity, stretching, and ordinary anti-inflammatory medications. Nothing really worked, so finally, out of desperation, I visited my doctor, who ordered some imaging.

Later, as my physician read the radiologist's report and gave me a sense of how serious the situation was, I saw in a flash of clarity that it was not my arthritis that had brought me to his office but my diseased ego. The shame and regret I felt about my behaviour that night in 2013 were mixed with some compassion – here, I have in mind the literal meaning of the word, which is "to suffer with" – for my sisters, my father, and my younger self of decades earlier.

Readers have read the rest of the story, which takes me to my first yoga class a few weeks later. However, there is a postscript.

Several months later, my teacher was helping me with padmasana (full lotus pose), which is done seated, with both ankles crossed over the opposite upper thighs. Many beginners cannot open their hips and bend their knees deeply enough to master this classic asana without pain. My teacher, Jack, sat in front of me to demonstrate the "full expression" of the posture and then to show me a "modification" that would help me to experience its key benefits (i.e., opening one's hips and improving posture) without pain. He could see me struggling to "get" even half lotus, with just one ankle resting in the hip crease of the opposite leg. I swore under my breath.

"What's wrong?" he asked.

I gestured at five or six other students around me, all of whom were comfortably seated in padmasana.

"*That*. Why can't I do *that*?" I whispered.

"Oh. And what if you *couldn't* do that?"

"What?? What do you mean?? Obviously, if I can't do *that*," I replied as I lifted my chin toward a former ballerina beside me in padmasana, "I'll never be able to do *that*," I said as I nodded in the direction of a twenty-eight-year-old graduate student in marichyasana D (ray of light pose, or pose of the sage Marichi D; see figure 3.3). This pose consists of a deep-seated twist with the right foot in half lotus, the right ankle in the left hip crease, the left knee bent toward the left shoulder, and the heel of the left foot situated near the left buttock; one twists one's torso to the left, reaching one's right arm around the outside of the left knee, and then bends the right arm and grasps the left hand, which reaches around the back as one looks to the back of the room.

Jack cocked his head, took a full breath, looked at me with great compassion, and repeated: "And what if you *couldn't* do that?"

He left me with this question. All the air emptied out of me. I uncrossed my legs and allowed my breathing to return to normal. I was disoriented and irritated. Why that smile? Why am I paying so much for rhetorical questions? Why bother if I could not make progress? As I settled myself into shavasana, something happened adjacent to my rational mind. I did not yet fully understand the connection between what had just occurred in the shala and what had happened that night on the soccer field several months before. But I sensed that my body was about to teach me.

Conclusion

Above, I noted that the students and teachers we met often referred not just to people such as van der Kolk and Maté but also to trauma-informed or trauma-sensitive yoga, therapy, pedagogy, leadership, and so forth. When I asked Braj, an Indian philosopher, what he thought about the central place of trauma talk in yogaland, he said that he appreciated that the many trauma-informed workshops, graduate degrees, teacher trainings, and websites respond to suffering and are part of a general critique of Western biomedicine. He also had no qualms with the idea that the body retains plenty of damage. Nonetheless, he expressed some impatience, noting that "this trauma-informed yoga talk is nonsense because you shouldn't inform your yoga by trauma. Your yoga should inform your trauma."

Here, he shifted the focus in a profound manner. Trauma-informed yoga is meant to sensitize practitioners to the fact that the body is keeping the

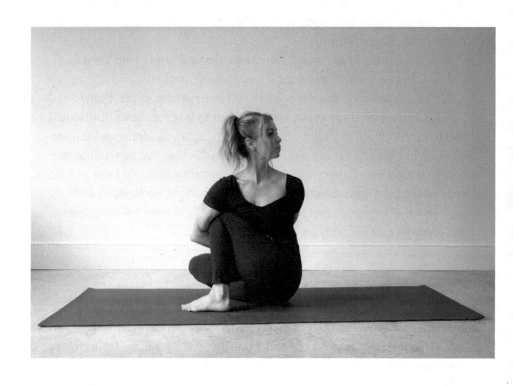

Figure 3.3
Marichyasana D (ray of light pose, or pose of the sage Marichi D)

score and that teachers therefore need to approach it with great care and deference but also with the knowledge that the body is the key to undoing damage that is impacting skin, digestion, joints, brain, mind, emotions, and more broadly the social world that so many damaged people inhabit.

However, what if you pursued the deeper – Braj would likely say classical or traditional Indic – benefits of yoga by going beyond the physical and aesthetic features of exquisite asanas? What if yoga was used explicitly as a means to see the contingent nature of all reality, the relationship between atman and Brahman, and the correct relationship between purusha and prakriti? What if the point of wearing flattering yoga clothes, paying a monthly membership fee, altering your social life, regularizing your sleeping habits, and practising asanas in a carefully curated room was not to look better or work the knots out of your lower back? What if you used these physical disciplines, spaces, and objects to understand the proper relationship between your finite self and the infinite universe of which you are – always and already – an integral part? Then, Braj's insight implies, traumatic events themselves might be transformed, might be experienced, perceived, and conceived differently, and perhaps might leave less of a mark on the body.

The challenge is that, as I observed during fieldwork, especially within nonlineage yoga contexts, there is a tension in Canadian and American yogalands between what one might call substantive and instrumental approaches to postural yoga, the latter being my own approach initially. In an instrumentalist model, yoga fixes damages – to mind and body – that happen in the normal course of surviving what Epstein calls "the trauma of everyday life."[45] The substantive approach is, as the word suggests, oriented toward a longer and richer relationship between a student and a community or style of practice. This perspective is most conducive to trauma therapy, which rejects the idea of quick fixes.[46]

Toward the end of my interviews, to learn about the ambitions of the most advanced practitioners – the teachers – I posed a hypothetical question. I asked whether they would feel that they had failed me as a student if I was still fixing one body part after another, five years after starting to work with them. The question was an effort to determine whether teachers hoped that students would eventually pursue the "higher" purposes, or angas (limbs), of the yoga system offered by Patanjali (i.e., breath work and advanced meditative techniques) or whether their main interest lay in coaxing Mary Oliver's soft animals into complex shapes.

To this hypothetical scenario, I received three kinds of responses. First, perhaps 20 per cent of teachers noted that since they bring up all (or at least many) of the limbs of yoga in their teaching, no student interested just in improving their bodies would be likely to tolerate their kind of teaching for more than a few weeks.

Second, most teachers (roughly 75 per cent) responded that if five years after I had begun working with them, I was moving from fixing my knees to fixing my lower back to fixing my weight, they would not feel that they or I had failed in any way. "I think it would just mean that is your karma," one teacher said. "I just take students one at a time and let them make choices about how to approach yoga," said another. One teacher noted, "Everyone has their own limits and interests, and if you were a body-oriented person, I would work with you this way."

Third, there were a few teachers, however, who said that they would be disappointed or who challenged the question itself. One teacher paused and looked at me askance. He could see the game in my question. "Yeah, I would think I had failed, if it was you," John said.

"Why if it's me?" I asked.

"Just because, not that I know you. But I know enough about you. Like I know you're smart, and [you] think, and [you like to] have conversations about stuff. And so if what I was teaching you in your yoga class had not spun out into your regular life in some way, then I would think I wasn't doing my job in some way. Maybe [for] someone else, it'd be good enough [but not for you]."

Another senior teacher, Jane, also saw through the question and responded to my scenario of looking only for physical fixes: "Well, I'm not sure I'd believe you." I was a bit shocked by her response. Why the doubt? Seeing my eyebrows shoot up, she added, "I feel like yoga works at different levels, and it works on those levels even without you knowing it … I think the reason you might be coming back time after time is not just because your ankle is feeling better or your knee is feeling better, but something about being in that room is giving you a deeper experience."

Whether or not teachers expect all students to take advantage of the full range of changes that yoga promises, the serious practitioners we met did not frame their asana practice as merely a means of improving flexibility and strength. Instead, as teachers and students advanced, asanas were typically understood as one part of an all-encompassing lifestyle, ethical system, disposition, and worldview in which traumatic suffering is neither avoided nor negated (since this is impossible anyway) but comes to sit more lightly in the body.

Readers familiar with the field of religious studies might recognize Bruce Lincoln's distinction between minimalist and maximalist orientations under the surface of this insight.[47] On the one hand, the maximalist approach to yoga – in which asanas, along with the other limbs of yoga, become the connective tissue of one's whole life – is typically what more advanced yogis have in mind when they speak of authentic or traditional yoga, or the yoga of Patanjali. On the other hand, the minimalist, or more casual and instrumental, relationship that occasional practitioners have with yoga is one that fits their practice into and "adds value to" their lifestyle, alongside other interests. I am not interested in determining the best or most authentic approach to postural yoga. That would differ for each practitioner, it seems to me. My own practice has become increasingly maximalist, but this orientation might work for me just because of my particular physical, economic, and psychological characteristics, and it might well change in the future. Regardless of where one might place oneself or someone else on this spectrum, the body is there, both keeping and settling the score. As Oliver puts it, "You only have to let the soft animal of your body love what it loves."

CHAPTER FOUR

Superpeople: From the Yoga *Sutras* to Yogaland

You should come to yoga. It's really great for core strength, flexibility,
and meeting women in their forties.
Sydney Fife (Jason Segel) in the film *I Love You, Man* (2009)

I do yoga now. I love it. I finally found an excuse to wear yoga pants everywhere.
Angela Ostrowski (Amy Poehler) in the film *Baby Mama* (2008)

I love jogging. It's like, you know, the only thing more boring and monotonous
than yoga.
Allison (Zooey Deschanel) in the film *Yes Man* (2008)

I do yoga. For the yoga, but mostly for the men.
Amy Redmond Mitchell (Mila Kunis) in the film *Bad Moms* (2016)

When newcomers step out of the world of a busy Brooklyn street and into
the anti-world of a Brooklyn studio, very few of them will be shocked by
what they encounter. Thanks to movies, sitcoms, magazines, and social
media, they will anticipate, and will usually experience, spaces that are clean,

well lit, airy, quiet, serene, vaguely Indic, and lightly scented, with carefully curated music playing softly. Perhaps the studio houses a wellness boutique with natural or (better yet) detoxifying deodorants, scents, and skin creams. There may be branded or (better yet) sustainably produced yoga clothes. There may be comfortable chairs and a vegetarian or (better yet) vegan cafe. Although newcomers might not notice, it is likely that studio owners will have made lighting, paint, and plumbing choices that are meant to render the space as yoga-friendly as possible.

Although yoga is often used in popular culture as a shorthand gesture to convey someone's shallowness, if one looks more closely, one will see that these spaces attain and retain their aura of gravitas and authenticity thanks to a certain kind of person. These individuals do things with their bodies that seem unimaginable for ordinary people, such as eka hasta vrikshasana (one-handed tree pose; see figure 4.1), parshva bakasana (side crow pose; see figure 4.2), or grasping the backs of their calves in urdhva dhanurasana (upward-facing bow pose; see figure 4.3). They perform these body- and mind-bending acts without looking even slightly taxed. I am not just describing serious seeker-students or asana practitioners – like myself, I suppose – but what we might call yoga jivanmuktas (superpeople). Whether these special teachers, students, or studio owners are there in the flesh or through images in real or digital yoga spaces, they are there – and they matter.

They are usually women. Also, they are usually white, radiantly healthy, and normally between twenty and forty, with flawless skin and neither visible body hair nor cellulite. They might have wrinkles or even grey hair, but both will be offset by an apparently effortless and yet exquisite hairstyle that is paired with a perfect scarf, earrings, ankle bracelets, or toe rings. Their posture is easy, erect, and strong. They appear to be in a state of constant readiness. You sense that they could be lawyers, painters, neurosurgeons, social workers, heiresses, stay-at-home mothers, models, or long-haul truckers. They could do anything.

They are well dressed in Lululemon, Alo Yoga, or equivalent brands.[1] When they show up on your social media feed or on yoga studio websites, they are on a beach or in a desert, a studio, a forest, or an Indian temple with an unclear connection to postural yoga. They are lit so well that you look in vain for evidence that they knew their picture was being taken. Of course, part of your mind is certain that these are staged photographs, but in another

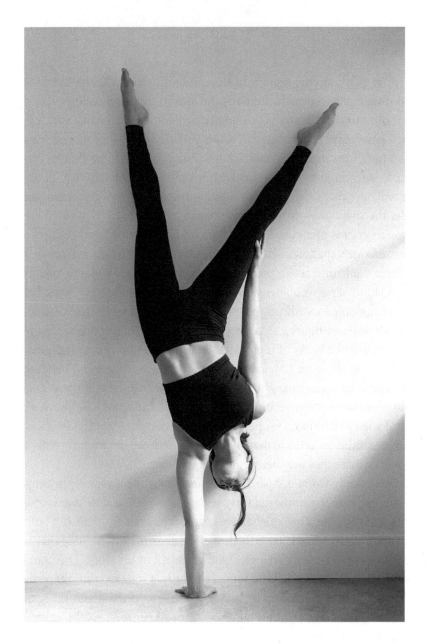

Figure 4.1
Eka hasta vrikshasana (one-handed tree pose)

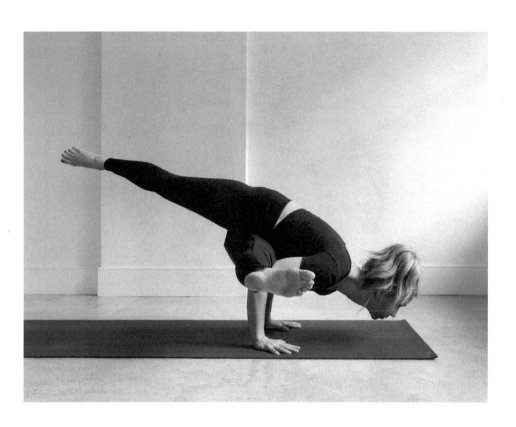

Figure 4.2
Parshva bakasana (side crow pose)

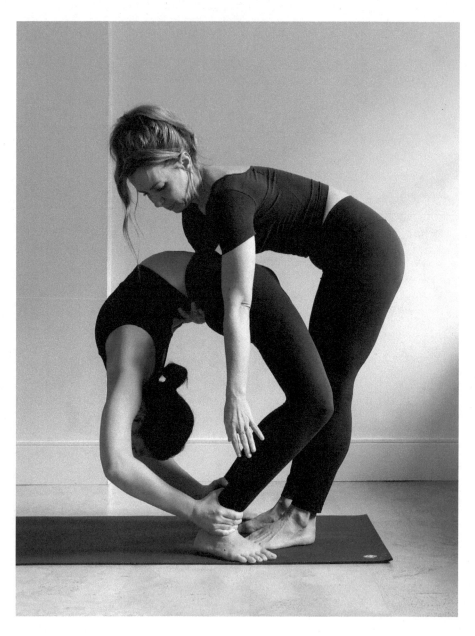

Figure 4.3

Urdhva dhanurasana (upward-facing bow pose)

part, you are enchanted, and it seems as though the image captures them in their natural resplendent perfection.

In the studio or in your social media feed, you may see a few male superhumans too. They are usually white and between roughly twenty-five and forty-five. They will sometimes be wearing a shirt but not usually, and one can hardly blame them. They will have flawless skin, often with artful tattoos. They will have excellent muscle definition, broad shoulders, and very minimal body hair.

For the people I have in mind, asana practice looks natural, enlivening, easy, and truly a reflection of their equanimity and vigour, and their verbal reflections on asana similarly reflect a calm confidence about the roots and purpose of yoga. In fact, their yoga has a preternatural – that is, outside of or beyond the natural – quality to it. This term is conceptually related to the idea of genius, at least in the sense that both words imply an extrarational or enchanted explanation or source for some experience or person.[2]

These superhumans are sometimes featured on the cover of major periodicals such as *Yoga Journal* and are the stars of most studios.[3] As I mentioned in the previous chapter, individual suffering is what often brings students into studios, but several have told me that when they arrived, they were enchanted by their studio's or their lineage's stars. The physical charisma of these accomplished yogis fills others with hopes for healthier, more attractive, less pain-wracked bodies. Without these luminous creatures, it is difficult to imagine the proliferation of commercially viable postural yoga (and its fairly standardized aesthetic) in North America, in much the same way that the viability of Hollywood is dependent on the vast appeal of its alluring superstars.

It is reasonable to focus on large systems such as capitalism and patriarchy to explain the ways that these figures have shaped the aesthetics and ethos of yogaland. Nonetheless, my sense is that beyond marketing and the relentless control of women's bodies in the service of capitalism, nationalism, white privilege, and patriarchy, something else is at work. There are forces within classical South Asian yoga itself, and within contemporary social theory, that might help us to understand the mystique not just of A-list "yogalebrities" but also of superhuman teachers, advanced students, and studio owners to whom modern postural yoga arguably owes its popularity.

In this chapter I suggest that yogaland is animated by jivanmuktas to a degree that commentators and practitioners have yet to explore adequately. This Sanskrit word is derived from the words jiva (life) and mukta (liberated), so the word is typically translated as "liberated while living," a concept in Vedanta philosophy that refers to rare people who attain moksha (liberation).[4] Although such a heightened state of consciousness is normally understood as enabling a person to escape samsara (the cycle of birth, death, and rebirth), jivanmuktas remain here, largely (or so the story goes) to help the rest of us. I am curious about the special creatures who inhabit and enchant the tangible and intangible spaces of North American yogaland. To be clear, I use the words superheroes, superhumans, siddhas (perfected beings), and jivanmuktas interchangeably, imprecisely, and playfully to capture the important roles that certain kinds of people play. Sanskrit experts may wince at my loose use of these terms. However, my account of these key figures is not grounded in their place in classical yoga texts and philosophy but in what I heard, observed, and felt during my fieldwork and throughout my time in yogaland.

Although the superpowers associated with advanced yogic practitioners are spelled out in detail in classical and medieval texts, it is the physical beauty and sex appeal of the modern exemplars that take centre stage in contemporary yogaland. However, their beauty is a necessary but not sufficient condition of their power and prestige among other students and teachers. That is, they do need to be physically appealing (within a fairly narrow set of norms), but their real impact is the product of the ways that their beauty somehow – magically, one might say – connotes optimal physical and ethereal qualities.[5]

In chapter 1 of this book, I described being momentarily seduced by the possibility that my svadharma (personal duty in the world) could somehow be connected to that of Swami Vivekananda. As exciting as a link between his life and both the Unitarian and Brahmin sides of my family story might have been, it is also entirely predictable that I would attribute an elaborate meaning to these facts. Just as I need to approach these coincidences with suspicion, I also need to guard against the tendency to wax poetic when it comes to jivanmuktas. I do not want to be beguiled by them, even though – to be honest – I find them beguiling.

The fact that, during my research and travels within yogaland, I have witnessed so many others being similarly smitten is just evidence that something interesting is at work in our minds and cultures, not that these figures uniquely merit attention. In my main field, religious studies, we are justifiably wary of any analysis that uses the categories and experiences of insiders without subjecting the categories and their personifications – the geniuses and siddhas – to rigorous scrutiny.[6] I quite agree with this wariness, and so I want to mute my own inclinations to stand in awe of these people and thereby avoid attributing all kinds of things to them beyond fortunate genetics and a strong capacity to commit themselves to training.

There is very little to be gained by placing such individuals in an intellectual black box that protects the special roles that they play and the privileges that they enjoy from ordinary inquiry. Whether these preternaturally gifted yogis are intrinsically unique – that is to say, whether they are *categorically* different from the rest of us – is something that I do not think can be determined. The point is that these figures are not just exalted within yogaland as accomplished individuals but also closely tied to the aesthetic norms idealized and pursued by others. Therefore, the question is how we might understand their importance and omnipresence in yogaland.

Perhaps I am making too much of these people. Perhaps their prominence in the actual or digitally mediated arenas of yogaland simply reflects that whatever else yoga might mean in contemporary North America, it is closely tied to styles (e.g., Iyengar, Ashtanga, Baptiste, Bikram, and Power yoga), clothing, mats, blocks, straps, workshops, online platforms, and retreats that are marketed to a very large cohort of consumers. It is no surprise that one finds images of physically fit and conventionally appealing people in yoga studios (and on yoga websites) since the most popular asana styles cater to strong, flexible, and balanced people with enough time and disposable income to join a studio.

Several studies, including two that I have conducted,[7] demonstrate empirically what many people know intuitively, namely that North American yoga students are relatively (although not exclusively) affluent, white, educated, and female. In our survey, 86 per cent of the participants were women, just under 20 per cent had an average household income above $200,000, and about 50 per cent had a master's degree or more. This profile will not come as a surprise to anyone who has spent any time observing yoga in North America (especially in the Iyengar and Ashtanga settings where many of my survey takers practice).

Obviously, a studio owner looking for an image for their website will choose something that they believe will appeal to their clients. Since beautiful people are more pleasing to look at than average-looking people – if you will forgive the tautology that conceals much about the ways that aesthetic standards are generated – we can expect to see an endless stream of such imagery through Facebook, TikTok, Twitter/X, and Instagram. Perhaps the prominence of such people in yoga spaces and yoga advertising is a straightforward business decision. If so, why complicate the matter?

Since most readers of this book are interested in peering behind the veil of North American yoga, I suspect that they will find this explanation quite unsatisfactory. A more critical approach to the beautiful and athletically gifted jivanmuktas would underline the many ways that they reflect the often problematic social and economic realities of the dominant society. Notably, the whiteness, affluence, femaleness, and conventional (and often intimidating) aesthetic standards in evidence in virtual and actual yoga studios reflect the power of exclusive norms and biases.[8]

For example, critics have noted the high cost of drop-in classes (about $20 to $30 per class) and of good yoga apparel (about $128 to $178 for Lululemon leggings), as well as the popularity of yoga among a relatively affluent cohort of (mostly) young to middle-aged able-bodied women with disposable income and free time.[9] It may be that yoga classes are often taken as part of a more affordable monthly membership package, that some studios offer donation-based and sliding-scale classes, and that drop-in classes are less expensive than personal training, physical therapy, and counselling sessions, but it is certainly true that yoga is not affordable for everyone.[10] Beyond the actual costs – however one calculates and compares them – the wellness aesthetic found in spas, yoga studios, and salons may convey an aura of affluence, privilege, and youthfulness that some would find alienating.

In addition to these real or imagined economic or class barriers, by now very few people would deny that many postural yoga communities – especially the ones with a younger target market such as those offering vinyasa and hot yoga – have tended both to celebrate a rather narrow beauty standard and potentially to exacerbate disordered eating habits.[11] Although some students and teachers (even many I have encountered in my own community) say that their practice helps them to deal with their anxiety, depression, and eating disorders,[12] the prominence of ultra-capable, youthful, (apparently) flawless, radiant teachers or senior students in studios, on websites, and on the walls of studios may also aggravate the problems. Obviously, these approaches to beauty and food are not specific to yoga but are symptoms of much larger societal trends.[13]

As well, it is important to note that most postural yoga spaces – here, I mean both brick-and-mortar as well as digital studios – are overwhelmingly white.[14] As a consequence, the superpowers that interest me in this chapter are most often associated with white practitioners. There are exceptions to this general rule – for example, Jessamyn Stanley and Laruga Glaser,[15] not to mention of course the Indian founders of several lineages – but the general whiteness of North American yogaland reflects the dominance of whiteness in North America.

I interviewed several African American teachers and studio owners in different cities, and they were all acutely aware of how unusual their roles were. Only one studio was serving mainly other racialized people, and in this New York case, the African Americanness of the teacher and the studio were central to the studio's offerings. The research assistant and I attended a class there (with about thirty-five others), and it was one of the only times that politics as well as riotous and often raunchy humour were front and centre. The space was decorated with both Indic as well as African art, and the banter between the teacher and many of the students was full of teasing, self-deprecation, and expletives that I have never heard in any other space that I have visited. My interview with the teacher revealed that her salty language, laid-back attitude, and cheeky repartee were tailored to appeal to her African American students. Only a few of the students – my research assistant and myself included – were not of African American background.[16]

The other African American teachers and owners we met taught mostly white students and were more recent additions to the yoga scene. They were clearly aware that they were outliers in yogaland. Jacob, an African American teacher in Brooklyn, explained that the low interest in yoga among his community had to do with cost as well as with the cultural stories around yoga in North America:

> There's always a stereotype [about yoga in the Black community], and there's always a stigma [associated with yoga]. Um, you know, white man's ice is colder ... To operate in a space, it does cost money. So you have to be able to create services that people can really afford, and they have to have disposable income. So when you look at this community, who is that? What type of people is that? That's not always Black people. It can be, but it's more of the new people coming into the community. And they can be white, Asian, uh, Hispanic, and the new Black people coming into the area that do not even understand about [the rich pre-gentrification history of this predominantly African American neighbourhood].[17]

The narrow aesthetic standards and racialized social class markers – such as hairstyles, tattoo types, decorating themes, and choices of clothing, mats, and vehicles – that clearly convey the community's boundaries are real, but it seems to me sensible to see them as effects of much larger forces. These standards and markers reflect the norms of a broader white-dominant, patriarchal ideology in which businesses profit not only from appealing to (and thereby creating) a clear target market of mostly white consumers with adequate disposable income but also from stirring up the anxieties of (mainly) women, many of whom push themselves relentlessly to get the toned body that they think is necessary for them to thrive both in the studio and in life.

It seems natural to focus on the ways that commercialized yoga in North America serves the interests of capitalism, patriarchy, and Orientalism or on the ways that the leaders in this community fetishize whiteness or unattainable lifestyles and physical standards. The evidence is strong, but this focus should not preclude other explanations not just for the magic that surrounds siddhas but also for the impact that they have on the aesthetics and ethos of yogaland.

First, however, let me consider some of the textual signposts on the road to contemporary yogaland that occur in the *Yoga Sutras*, with the corresponding numbers of the sutras indicated in parentheses.

One of my dogs is a semi-feral beagle-Catahoula mix. Her piercing and yet indifferent stare leaves me with a deep wish to be able to understand her thoughts. Perhaps her cognition would be limited to "Give me a treat" or "You smell weird." However, it seems that there is a depth to her that I could fathom only by being able to apprehend her language.

Speaking of unfamiliar languages, when I feel adrift in another country, I often dream that I can converse fluently in Hindi, Japanese, Catalan, or German (3.17).

I am not generally convinced that anyone lives more than a single life, but on the days when this possibility does not seem preposterous, I wish that I might glimpse my former lives (3.18).

From time to time, I find someone so baffling that I wish I could "get inside their minds." The ability to know the mind of another would certainly enable me to avoid misunderstandings and to enrich myself (3.19).

I wish that I was as strong as an elephant. That would make it much easier to do yard work and to change flat tires (3.25). I am currently not able to be everywhere, so I would love to have ultra-sensitive perceptual abilities that would allow me to see and know things anywhere in the universe (3.26).

I sometimes lose track of galaxies, and I have some common health anxieties, so I would appreciate knowing the position of the stars in the sky (3.28), the current situation of my body (3.30), and the time of my death (3.23).

While I am cataloguing my wishes, I should note that I would also like to be able to:

- change into another species (3.2)
- overcome hunger and thirst (3.31)
- see siddhas (perfected beings) (3.33)
- attain divine faculties of seeing, hearing, touch, taste, and smell (3.37)
- enter the body of another person at will (3.39)
- walk on water or levitate (3.40)

- hear distant and divine sounds (3.42)
- fly (3.43)

I have taken some liberties, but depending on which interpretation of the *Yoga Sutras* one reads, one will have come across these special powers.[18]

Patanjali's *Yoga Sutras* is sometimes called "the bible of yoga," which is accurate at least in the sense that the text is certainly quite central in the discussion of classical and modern yoga. As well, people attribute all manner of claims to the *Yoga Sutras* that are not really (or indisputably) in the text. The text is the subject of innumerable workshops, courses, websites, books, and articles; it is a book often owned if not always carefully studied by practitioners and studio owners; and the authorship, meaning, and divine inspiration of the text are disputed.

Beyond that, the Christian Bible and the *Yoga Sutras* are quite dissimilar. The 196 short sutras (from the Sanskrit word for "threads") typically include the original Sanskrit sutra, a direct translation, and then much longer "glosses" or explanations and interpretations by the sage Vyasa, who is possibly Patanjali himself; in many editions, the sutras, translations, and initial glosses are followed by the additional interpretations of, for example, B.K.S. Iyengar, Swami Satchidananda Saraswati, Swami Vivekananda, or some other interlocutor. For many centuries, the text had a mostly scholarly readership and was in a sense repopularized as the central expression of yoga largely by Vivekananda, which occurred only in the late nineteenth and early twentieth centuries.[19]

Enthusiastic yogis often buy a copy and expect to read about the connection between asana practice and ancient Indic philosophy and psychology. Many people do not get past the first two padas (chapters), by which point they either feel overwhelmed by the powerful compression of the sutras or discover that there is virtually nothing said in the book about the asanas that one might see in most studios.

All that the text has to say about physical postures appears in sutras 2.46, 2.47, and 2.48, in which – to abbreviate a longer, more interesting conversation – yogis are instructed to sit in a posture (the "as" in "asana" means "to sit") that is firm and pleasant and to meditate on the infinite. Popular yoga writer Stephen Cope notes that the asana that Patanjali likely has in mind is padmasana (full lotus pose) or some variation of it. There are no instructions in the text for trikonasana (triangle pose; see figure 4.4), shirshasana (headstand pose; see figure 4.5), badha konasana (bound angle pose; see figure 4.6), or any of the other common asanas associated with modern postural practice. This is not to say that the body and its discipline were not important to Patanjali and to the larger oral tradition of his era but only that asana instruction was not the author's central concern.[20] The psychospiritual benefits and broader philosophical framework of yoga seem to have been his main interest.

This is not the place – nor am I the person – to reflect extensively on the intentions of Patanjali or on the structure or content of the *Yoga Sutras* themselves. I juxtapose the very few (and very vague) references to asanas with the many (and often relatively detailed) references to special powers for two reasons. First, I want to note how curious it is that so little is made in yogaland of the mind reading, shape-shifting, flying, omniscience, and invisibility that are promised or attributed to advanced yogis. When I mentioned the special powers during interviews and focus groups, as well as anywhere else that I travelled in yogaland, people mostly laughed awkwardly and changed the subject, usually gesturing to the idea that siddhis (special powers) are associated with the more esoteric and advanced levels of practice. As Ruth, a teacher in Toronto, said, "I mean, even if you're just looking at like the eight limbs [described in the *Yoga Sutras*], you get into some trippy stuff. I almost feel like I can read that [third] pada and I can understand it, but I won't be able to truly grasp any of the special powers stuff until I've been practising for my whole life. And so I don't feel as connected to that kind of thing as I do to the first couple of chapters."

Perhaps these powers are downplayed because as Edwin Bryant observes in *The Yoga Sutras of Patanjali* (2009), "That the *siddhis* are potential impediments to the goal of *yoga* is a widespread position in Indic traditions."[21] In sutra 3.38 of the *Yoga Sutras*, Patanjali himself warns, "These [*siddhis*] are obstacles to *samadhi* [meditative absorption]; but they are powers in the worldly state."[22] In *Light on the Yoga Sutras of Patanjali* (1993), Iyengar notes, "The yogi may mistake these accomplishments and rewards for the end and aim of yogic practices."[23] The siddhis are framed as worldly consequences, but not objectives, of advancement within a larger system involving one's

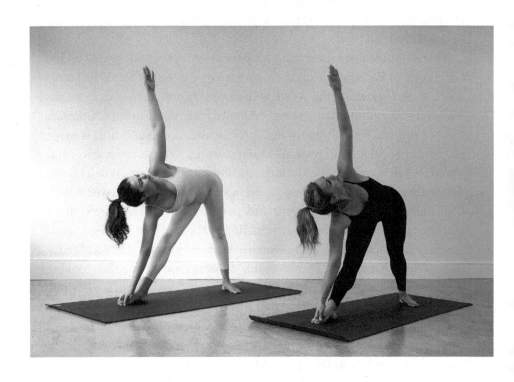

Figure 4.4
Trikonasana (triangle pose)

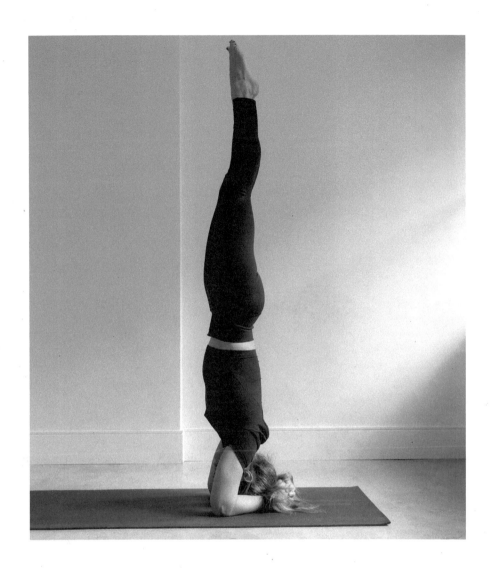

Figure 4.5
Shirshasana (headstand pose)

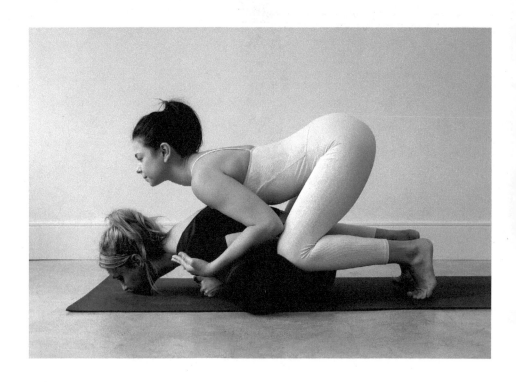

Figure 4.6

Badha konasana (bound angle pose)

ethical behaviour (the first two limbs of Patanjali's eight-limbed system), as well as asanas, pranayama (breath work), and meditative practices.

Nonetheless, even if we accept the argument that siddhis are rarely discussed in yogaland because Patanjali and those who followed him wanted to discourage distractions, it is hard to understand the development of yoga in South Asia, and elsewhere, without them.[24] As Mark Singleton and James Mallinson make clear in their landmark study *Roots of Yoga* (2017),[25] for much of the long history of yoga, there has been a great interest among practitioners in techniques and practices that would aid the quest for immortality, transcendence, occult abilities, and the capacity to retain or direct life energies. For example, there are techniques focused on kundalini (the coiled serpent of energy) said to live at the base of the spine and those focused on bindu (the point where creation begins and is unified), usually identified with semen and thought to gather in the head. We also see these pursuits in the less popular but far more asana-oriented fifteenth-century *Hatha Yoga Pradipika* by Svatmarama, the third premodern text, after the *Bhagavad Gita* and the *Yoga Sutras*, that one might find in the lending libraries of North American studios.

Finally, in the best-selling *Autobiography of a Yogi* (1946) by Paramahansa Yogananda, the author reflects on the nature of the ancient traditions of Kriya Yoga, a variety of physical and esoteric practices designed to achieve mastery over one's body, and on their value to him and others within the history of yoga. Yogananda's book was a massive success – with people such as Steve Jobs, George Harrison, Ravi Shankar, and Andrew Weil citing it as a major influence on their lives – because of the power of Kriya Yoga to help one master, overcome, or transform one's body so that it might be a site or tool of one's own liberation.[26]

In contemporary Western societies that lack the public presence of monastics, not to mention wandering ash-covered sadhus (ascetics),[27] special yogic powers have become associated with gifted practitioners who are the standard-bearers of beautiful digital or actual studios and who offer workshops in picturesque retreat settings or as part of spiritual travel excursions to India.[28] Although these gifted yogis need to use language and imagery that communicate the ineffable power of their offerings – and of themselves as conduits of yoga's transformative potential – the message will often be embedded in familiar themes related to powerful Western perspectives on individualism, wellness, and the dominant scientific paradigm.

Consider this example. The project research assistant and I met with Toni, a significant figure in US yogaland – and a jivanmukta, in my opinion – on the large deck adjacent to a studio that she built fifteen years earlier with friends in Rolling Hills Estates, southwest of Los Angeles. We sat on cushions covered in tapestries and appreciated the views of the ocean through the palm trees that surrounded the studio. Well educated and originally from France, she spoke in a voice that still carried the music of her native language. She offered us tea and figs from her studio garden, which we enjoyed as we talked and admired the hummingbirds visiting the many plants flowering on the deck.

Toni, in her late forties, was impeccably dressed that day in a pure white bodysuit over which she had draped a sheer grey linen scarf. Her auburn hair was cut short, and she wore neither makeup nor jewellery.

I found myself adjusting my hips on the floor cushion throughout the interview, partly because I am an office denizen in my mid-fifties who is not used to sitting on the ground and partly because I was stiff from practising so much in recent months. Toni, in contrast, exuded grace and confidence and sat almost perfectly still for an hour and a half. We spoke of her large family in France, her time spent as a painter and dancer in Barcelona, and her eventual move to Los Angeles to pursue modelling and yoga teaching. When the conversation turned to the special powers promised in the yoga tradition, Toni introduced the idea of quantum physics (and was not the only one to do so):

Quantum physicists talk about the world upon world upon worlds. It's exactly what they speak about in the third pada [of the *Yoga Sutras*, where most of the powers are delineated] – the world upon world upon worlds and all the special powers. I mean ... in the quantum realm, of course, you can move from one location to another. You could bilocate or you can read people['s minds]; you can transcend the ordinary capacities of the mind. You can transcend the ordinary secretions of the glandular system and access psychedelic realms with your own inner pharmacy. That, to me, is everything that's spoken of in the third pada.

And so I feel like human beings [are] on this evolutionary journey, and since science is finally catching up with this ancient tradition [of yoga], like, wow, what's possible for us? Because to me, if you can believe it, you can do it. We know this from the practice [of yoga]. If you can believe you can do a handstand, you can do a handstand.

The research assistant shared my impression: Toni was enthralling. In her presence, time seemed to pass differently. We left her home rather reluctantly, I confess, and were briefly speechless as we drove away, with the first words in the car being "What just happened?" But we were both too disoriented to remember afterward who posed this question. So it goes in the meeting of ordinary people and siddhas.

These gifted practitioners excel not just in beauty and strength. It is my sense that among many of the people I met in yogaland, their physical and aesthetic endowments are understood to be the outward manifestations of a jivanmukta's internal and essential distinction from ordinary people. The fact that not everyone has access to these powers confers great spiritual and worldly prestige upon those who do. More than that, however, these kind, graceful, and accomplished yogis glow with a light that can illuminate others in their communities. (Earlier, I promised to resist this kind of exalted rhetoric. Forgive me, but without rhapsodic language, it is hard to capture the impact of these people on those around them, myself included.)

A great many of us say that we do not believe in magic, but secretly, subtly, or subconsciously, most of us do. We see this belief when we consider the impact of a siddha's practice and persona.

During fieldwork in Toronto, I went out for dinner with some old friends. As we were all catching up after a decade apart, we shared stories about our respective middle-aged life situations: divorces, aging parents, difficult health predicaments, empty nests, new jobs, pets, and houses.

A few of us shared some acquaintances within the yoga world and began to update one another about their lives. One such shared friend is Allie, a model and gifted yoga teacher with an impeccable practice.

Several people have commented to me that when she enters a room, those already there can feel a change in the composition of the air. Everyone – women, men, children – seems to be captivated by her, even when she is just minding her own business. Several women I know have said that they sometimes have to look away from her when they are in conversation because, otherwise, they struggle to concentrate. She and her husband have three children and live in an elegant home in Ontario. When her name came up in conversation, a friend winced and told us that Allie's daughter had just died suddenly from a cardiac condition that no one knew existed.

Everyone at the table gasped at this news. After a pregnant pause, one of our friends, Rob, said, "Oh my God, this is awful. Allie has everything – she is so perfect, beautiful children, a stunning practice, magazine-ready house, wonderful husband, everything was perfect. You just never expect terrible things to happen to people like her."

People like her. The table was silent for a moment, struck by Rob's comment. It was certainly gauche, but it was also an honest articulation of something that many of us were thinking or feeling but that no one else dared to say. Another way to put it would have been: "But Allie is magic. Why wouldn't she and those she loved be protected by the special force that clearly surrounds her?"

The German historian and sociologist Max Weber is most famous for *The Protestant Work Ethic and the Spirit of Capitalism* (1904), in which he outlined the power of religious ideas to act as "switchmen" in important moments of social change. An equally important contribution that he made to our shared intellectual life was his work on charisma (from the Greek word meaning "favour, gift, or grace"). Charismatic authority is based on an individual's special power to draw others to them and to compel or impel them to act in a manner not based on tradition (i.e., it has always been done this way) or reason (i.e., it is sensible to do it this way) but on the leader's will (i.e., they inspire us to do it this way). This is not to say that charismatic figures do not also appeal to reason, and it is not to say that followers entirely lose their agency around such people. It is simply the case that such individuals – like the magical Allie – are thought to be unique, and their gifts often animate groups.

It is often – indeed, usually – the case that charismatic authority is a key feature of political and social movements. In some cases, this kind of authority is the sine qua non of such transformative groups. Consider Malcolm X, Martin Luther King, Mohandas Gandhi, or the Tibetan Buddhist leader Trungpa Rinpoche, four charismatic leaders who led movements that had significant impacts on the societies in which they lived. Speaking of Trungpa Rinpoche, one devotee remarked, "There was a kind of honey in his being,"[29] a comment that captures well the power not just of this eccentric figure but also of charisma itself.

The Indian yoga world has its charismatic figures too. Among these figures are people such as Swami Vivekananda, Swami Sivananda, Paramahansa Yogananda, Maharishi Mahesh Yogi, Sadhguru, Tirumalai Krishnamacharya, and his students Pattabhi Jois and B.K.S. Iyengar, the last two being responsible for inspiring much of twentieth-century postural practice in North America.[30] Each of these men has an important place in the fascinating story of contemporary yoga – both in India and abroad.[31] Movements have emerged around these individuals, with ashrams, training facilities, publication houses, yoga brands, resorts, journals, and so on.

As is typical of charismatic figures, stories circulate about their special abilities, such as the claim that Yogananda's body did not decay in the normal way after he died and the claim that Bikram Choudhury needs almost no sleep.[32] Even people in nonlineage hatha yoga communities – core, power, vinyasa, flow, and Yin – speak of these people, especially Krishnamacharya, with reverence.

I am concerned here not with these individual legendary twentieth-century teachers, about whom much has already been written,[33] but with the ways that the Weberian notion of charisma helps to explain the power that accrues to many twenty-first-century postural yoga teachers and adepts, whether one is exposed to them personally or through YouTube, Instagram, Facebook, or TikTok.

To be clear, not all famous teachers or even advanced students possess charisma or wield charismatic authority (or else it would not be special). Nevertheless, there is a powerful aura surrounding those North American teachers and students who radiate strength, beauty, and health and whose clothes, hairstyles, diets, transformative experiences in India, and capacity to tell a story or chant a mantra with passable Sanskrit pronunciation set them apart. There is a kind of magic in these luminous, lithe creatures who can move effortlessly from shirshasana (headstand pose) to urdhva padma-sana (upward lotus pose; see figure 4.7), which requires balancing on one's shoulders and on the back of one's head, to matsyasana (fish pose; see figure 4.8). It is hard to look away from their enchanted choreography.

With Weber's charismatic authority in mind, it should come as no surprise that it is common to think – perhaps, more accurately, to feel – that jivanmuktas and even their loved ones are somehow blessed and ought to be immune to heart attacks, unburdened by poor choices, and undaunted by serious physical and moral challenges. That is certainly magical thinking, but it is common precisely because such beguiling people seem somehow set apart, even sanctified, which gives them tremendous personal and social power.

Are they treated in this manner because of something inherently special about them, or does the special treatment that they receive reflect a deep need in our society for enchanted people to embody our higher ideals and to relieve us of the burden of being small, vulnerable creatures in an indifferent world? I am inclined to think the latter, but I also recognize the tendency in me – a weakness, perhaps – to feel surprised, even betrayed, when siddhas behave in ordinary and even disappointing ways.

It is also quite understandable that siddhas such as Toni would have a high confidence in the key lessons of quantum physics. Clearly, many yogis (and others intrigued by alternative and complementary modes of healing) interpret quantum physics as confirming their hopes for a more enchanted, holistic world that is not just the product of crass and predictable social forces.[34] A yoga student I met at a workshop told me that she had chosen to move from Europe to a particular US city without having any knowledge of the city. Her move was based on intuition, she said. I pressed her for some more context for this feeling; I suspected that she must have had at least some knowledge about the new city and some sense that her intuition was worth heeding. She explained,

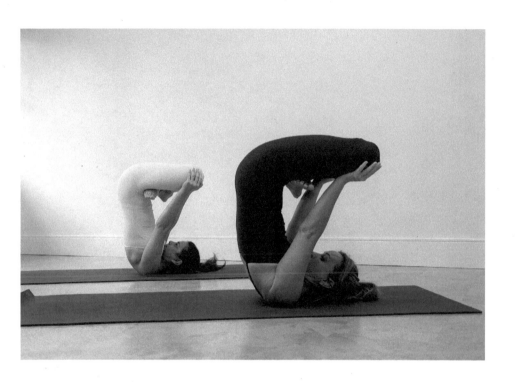

Figure 4.7
Urdhva padmasana (upward lotus pose)

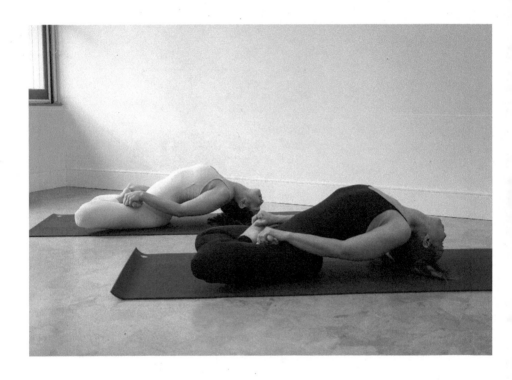

Figure 4.8
Matsyasana (fish pose)

I think I see what you're asking, but that question comes out of the Newtonian imagination. But if you are thinking along the lines of quantum physics, a thing can be both here and there. What we think of as ourselves and our imaginations are basically just made up, and so of course it is not at all impossible for me to have knowledge about this city without "knowing" anything or doing any "research" about it. I am not limited by the Newtonian account of time and space, so I can understand things without having what a Newtonian person would think of as direct experience of them.[35]

Whether trained physicists would recognize quantum mechanics in the ways that yogis represent it is another question entirely, but it is clear that for yogis – siddhas and others I have met – the appeal of this complex branch of science lies in its promise to offer the "post-Newtonian" worldview that Toni said would allow us all to "transcend the ordinary capacities of the mind" and to activate our "own inner pharmacy" since "if you can believe it, you can do it." Whether special powers allow us to avoid illness, understand the language of our peculiar pets, sit for hours in padmasana, clasp one's ankles in a deep backbend, or traverse time and space, they are essential features of yogaland.

Conclusion

Yoga is often a punchline in North American popular culture – and for good reason. Throughout yogaland, one does not need to look very hard to see harmful body ideals and people attracted to the practice for the superficial reasons sketched in this chapter's opening Hollywood quips. Of course, in addition, there are troubling affinities between yoga and Orientalism, cultural appropriation, white supremacy, and conspiracy theories.[36] But when we look beyond these common (and fair) criticisms, we find some exceptional people: preternaturally gifted, strong, conventionally gorgeous, flexible, corporeally intelligent, articulate students and teachers. These individuals are giants in yogaland – which I mean almost literally, in the sense that they seem to occupy a disproportionate amount of symbolic, actual, and digital space compared with regular students and teachers.

I have been intentionally nonspecific in the way that I identify them. I could name some obvious examples,[37] but I do not think it is helpful to focus our attention on celebrities. My sense is that beyond the charismatic founders and current stars of yogaland, there are people in every city, likely in every studio community, whose gifts set them apart. Some of them are hardly known outside of their studios or cities; some of them are known only through social media. But wherever they are, whenever they practice, they shine, and their charismatic power influences the ethos and aesthetics of yogaland.

I outlined the siddhis promised in the *Yoga Sutras* to indicate that it is not only neoliberalism, the fashion industry, white supremacy, and patriarchy that explain why certain kinds of people are so often featured as models, teachers, and leaders. In addition to the plausible ideological explanations for the roles of such people within yogaland, it is worthwhile to consider the power of texts such as the *Yoga Sutras* and charisma as well.

People rarely speak of them, but I suspect that these special powers are crucial features of postural yoga's success both in South Asia and in contemporary North America, just as the allegedly supernatural power of the saints, martyrs, and angelic figures within Christianity are surely not unrelated to its reach throughout Western history. During the development of yoga, however, writers from Patanjali to B.K.S. Iyengar to Edwin Bryant to my own teachers have warned against a fixation on the siddhis. This ancient and enduring caution reflects an awareness of the projections and manipulations that predictably come into play once a "sacred text" or a "bible of …" can be invoked to justify for oneself or one's teachers an exemption from ordinary moral or physical limits.

Throughout the history of yoga, the origin and uses of these special powers – who gets them, how they ought to be used, whether they are an end or a means – are articulated in ways that reflect the communities in which the text is nested. Solo renunciants, groups of Nath warrior-ascetics, Brahmin householders, and princes determined to get along with a new imperial presence have their own predictably distinctive approaches to the definition, origin, value, and use of siddhis.[38]

When postural yoga began to flourish in North America in roughly the 1980s, it was not at all surprising that the special powers articulated in the *Yoga Sutras* did not get much attention. After all, the new yoga teachers and students were economically comfortable people (mostly women) who were devoted to self-improvement, a preoccupation that neoliberalism made necessary; who were enthusiastic about the wisdom of Asia, which retained its perennial allure even when the dominant forms of Christianity began to decline; who were seeking some sacred source for their incipient power at a time when women finally, if also fitfully, were granted greater economic and sexual liberation; and who were not greatly concerned about cultural appropriation, which is a concern of a small group of people in any case.[39]

My sense is that over the past thirty or forty years, most North American yoga students and teachers would have been uncomfortable with the list of special powers that I provided above but might also have had experiences of bodily empowerment through their yoga practice. This empowerment would have been especially appealing for students burdened by trauma or exposure to a repressive form of Christianity. They may also have had a taste of samadhi through one or another yogic practice, which would have been especially appealing for the children and grandchildren of the 1960s raised to value mysticism, individualism, and free-spiritedness. Or perhaps they enjoyed the experience of being part of a community that (to use another Weberian term) "routinized" the special powers attributed to their founders. This experience would have been especially appealing for people alienated by suburbanization, individualism, and the loneliness that, according to American sociologist Robert Putnam, leads people to "bowl alone" as opposed to joining a league.[40]

The general silence around what we might call the siddhi sutras – which, I should reiterate, greatly outnumber the asana sutras in Patanjali's text – suggests that siddhis might have been sublimated when postural yoga expanded rapidly in North America. In confident, Protestant-dominated, scientifically oriented societies such as the United States and Canada, where teachers (understandably) needed to emphasize the nonreligious, nonexotic health benefits of postural yoga, the extravagant powers promised in the *Yoga Sutras* – and also in the *Hatha Yoga Pradipika* and in the broader yogic tradition – became rather "cringe-worthy" due to their "trippy" qualities, to use the language of a teacher we interviewed in Toronto. Nonetheless, these powers and these powerful people have continued to enchant yogaland.

All things considered, it would be understandable if Western yogis were to experience the picturesque teachers, students, and models who have floated through this chapter as embodiments of hope for the way that an enchanted life might look, move, and feel.

Of course, as so much of the research on modern postural yoga demonstrates, the local and global stars of yogaland are certainly enmeshed in patriarchy, capitalism, and Orientalism.[41] My experience and research certainly confirm this finding. Beyond this circumstance, however, Patanjali and Weber enrich our understanding of why a particular practitioner in San Antonio, Moncton, or Miami might be held in such high esteem and why people want to stare at them and cannot think of them as entirely mortal. My sense is that the power of such people is not only a function of old (yet timeless) promises made in texts such as the *Yoga Sutras* but also a testament to the raw charismatic magnetism of physical splendour and athletic prowess. The power that they embody is not just personal but also social. The siddhas who grace yoga spaces provide ordinary practitioners with ideals of finesse, awareness, and strength, while promoting solidarity within communities inspired by a shared sense of nearly infinite human potential.

In the next chapter, I explore two crises. The first came to light when critics and practitioners learned that some of the founders and leaders in the postural yoga world had used their social and special powers to take advantage of their students. The second came to light when critics and practitioners started to appreciate the extent to which yogaland has irresponsibly borrowed South Asian religious and cultural resources. At the heart of these difficulties, we find a luminous, beguiling, eternal, charismatic India.

CHAPTER FIVE

The Centre Held: Yoga after #MeToo and Cultural Appropriation

Do you remember the dolphins in the canals of Venice in the spring of 2020? Did you feel, as I did, a sense of hope when social media showed those dorsal fins cut through the water, with the sound of exultant Italians in the background? Sadly, stories about the "rewilding" of cities during the pandemic were mainly debunked,[1] although I assume that most readers will remember why the prospect of global healing seemed so desirable.

A few years later, the losses of that period (including roughly 7 million people) haunt many of us. Of course, the trauma was intensified by the coincidence of several other events or social forces: the political tumult in the United States, Canada, and other societies as they tilted toward authoritarianism; inadequate responses to our climate emergency; slow progress on Indigenous reconciliation in Canada; growing levels of income inequality; and violence and harassment against women rendered conspicuous in the #MeToo movement. The COVID-19 pandemic was just one of the portentous political and public health events that some call a "polycrisis" or "syndemic."[2]

The words of the poet William Butler Yeats, written in the aftermath of the First World War, are quoted so often that they seem banal, but they capture fears that people have about our current moment:

Turning and turning in the widening gyre
The falcon cannot hear the falconer;
Things fall apart; the centre cannot hold;
Mere anarchy is loosed upon the world,
The blood-dimmed tide is loosed, and everywhere
The ceremony of innocence is drowned;
The best lack all conviction, while the worst
Are full of passionate intensity.

The centre cannot hold, and the best lack all conviction. One could hardly be faulted for hoping the Venetian dolphins were harbingers of a better world.

The yoga world is in the midst of its own syndemic, incorporating the economic impact of the pandemic, the crises associated with sexual misconduct scandals, and the heightened sensitivities that have emerged around cultural appropriation.

Yogaland has its own dolphins, its own real and imagined promises. Scholars and critics might doubt whether yoga's benefits are deep or long-lasting, and we might observe the many ways that the features of the world persist in the anti-world of a studio. Nonetheless, the senior teachers and students we met seemed certain that they had an antidote to a loud, fast, and dirty world that had become so difficult during the larger syndemic.

Of course, the basic promises made by yoga studios appeal to so many people because, usually, they are attainable: over time, you can walk without pain, touch your toes, breathe more deeply, lose weight, and sleep better. Although this healing was the kind that I was seeking when I hobbled into my first yoga class in my baggy old sweatpants, other people are drawn into studios by reports that yoga will deliver profound psychological, philosophical, or spiritual benefits. These pursuits are often achievable too: you might get along better with friends and family, improve your ability to concentrate, develop more compassion for others, begin a regular meditation practice, or grasp, even momentarily, your place within a larger reality.

Do newcomers to yogaland seek definitive medical evidence for the effectiveness of postural yoga? Generally, no. It certainly is the case that the existing scientific data seem to be moving slowly in the direction of a consensus about the positive impacts of postural yoga.[3] As exciting as this outcome might be for people eager to post the headlines of studies on social media accompanied by a smug "Told you so" comment, most committed practitioners pay very little attention to scientific evidence rooted in Western or Indic paradigms.[4]

If students are generally neither looking for nor very fussy about randomized, double-blind peer-reviewed validations of yoga, are they drawn in by the intellectual coherence of the religious or philosophical paradigm that undergirds yoga practice? Some people certainly love this part of the backstory of yoga, and there are innumerable outlets for such an orientation,[5] but this focus is not the dominant appeal of the practice for students either.

The yoga teachers we met said that virtually all of their students begin yoga to improve their physical or mental well-being. Some are also, or eventually become, passionate about the philosophical or spiritual aspects of a postural practice, but of course very few will pursue this focus formally.[6]

However, this is not to say that there are no other common concerns, ideas, values, or practices that bind yoga practitioners together. I have discussed the ways postural yoga may be viewed as a complementary medical intervention, a response to trauma, a meeting place of magic and charisma, or a means of escaping or challenging the political status quo.

But there is another important element of yoga spaces that newcomers and scholars will likely notice. In the anti-world of Canadian and American studios, the regular world is intentionally subverted, tamed, beautified, and reordered, all with the help of India, a real and imagined place or even state of mind. Academics might say that India is a "polysemic signifier," which is a somewhat pretentious way to say that, just like concepts such as wellness, the West, health, happiness, and beauty, India means and points to a wide variety of things. There is no referee available to determine what we can and should say about India (although many people in yogaland claim to be able to do exactly that), but there is no doubting the power of India as a symbol. As Sunila S. Kale and Christian Lee Novetzke write,

Although India is not the financial or demographic hub of MPY [modern postural yoga], India and Indian culture remain key markers of authenticity in the global practice of yoga today. MPY privileges Indian cultural forms, like Sanskrit and Indian music (or facsimiles of Indian music), in such a way as to invest these things with the cultural capital of "authenticity." The founding gurus and many of the current leaders of MPY are Indian, and the commodity sign of Indian-ness remains a key element of yoga branding, from the use of Sanskrit words like "namaste," "mantra," and "om" to images easily identified with India (designs, motifs, the color saffron, Hindu deities, Sanskrit words, etc.). And it is still a requirement in almost all yoga training courses in America to study the classical texts of yoga, such as Patanjali's *Yogasūtras* and the *Haṭha Yoga Pradīpikā*.[7]

As I sat in the foyer of an established studio in Toronto, an advanced practitioner captured this aspect of India's symbolic power perfectly. "Without what India has given us, all we're doing is exercise," he said. Following his lead, I am interested here not in the history or politics of South Asia but in India as a powerful idea on which North American yoga spaces rely either implicitly or explicitly.

Even people who have never set foot on the subcontinent already know that India is the home of yoga; they know that serious students and teachers are either expected to go there or to want to do so. Religious studies colleagues would say that India is a crucial component of the "authorizing discourse" or "plausibility structure" of North American yogaland.[8] Whether practitioners are talking about a beloved ashram, the insights of a revered guru, their own Sanskrit tattoos, their dietary practices, or their effort to pronounce invocations correctly, allusions or direct references to India convey gravitas to lineages, styles, teacher-training programs, teachers, and devoted students.

The particular significance of India is arguably best apprehended when it is under siege, as has been the case in recent years thanks to yoga's own syndemic. I focus both on the sexual scandals that rocked yogaland and on the effort to grapple with cultural appropriation. What impact have these two deeply disruptive experiences had on the idea of India, this load-bearing wall of North American yoga? Through interviews, a survey, focus groups, site visits, and years of practice and travel in yogaland, I was surprised to discover that these two tribulations, which could have drowned what Yeats might have called postural yoga's "ceremony of innocence," have not destroyed it. In the following pages I reflect on these tribulations and the reasons why yoga seems to survive.

Don't Fight the Yoga

Before we consider these two difficult periods in contemporary postural yogaland, it would be helpful to reflect more on the Indic features of so many yoga spaces. Of course, there are the easy examples: the music playing in the lobby, incense, posters, tattoos, the teacher-training credentials mentioned in promotional material,[9] often-garlanded photos of Indian gurus, statues of Ganesh, Shiva, and Buddha, posters for events in support of Indian social issues such as Yoga Gives Back, and advertisements for retreats, tours, and workshops in Rishikesh, Pune, Goa, or Mysore.

These are, however, not the only ways that India – the idea more than the state – makes its presence known in yogaland. As I have noted, the project research assistant and I took sixty-five yoga classes in Victoria, Indianapolis, Winnipeg, Toronto, New York, Los Angeles, and Vancouver. Our classes augmented the survey, the hundreds of classes that we had taken before and after the project, and my teacher-training experience. My understanding of India – both as a metaphor (or map) and as an actual country (or territory) – is also inflected by my own mixed ethnic background and by my visit there two years before I took up a serious yoga practice. So India was present in my mind in a variety of ways, as a sound or an echo, offering an alternative to the cacophony of North America.

An experience I had during fieldwork highlights the often subtle influence of Indian ways of being in North America's yogaland. The story is rooted in one of our research sites, but it conveys a distinctive social order evident in many of the lineage-based spaces that I have visited over the years.

One day in New York, in the middle of an Ashtanga class of about fifteen students,[10] I performed what I thought was a solid "jump-back" and "jump-through" vinyasa combination.[11]

The jump-back and jump-through are important transitional moves that begin when one is seated with shins lightly crossed, knees drawn in toward the chest, and hands flat on the mat beside the hips. One breathes in while lifting oneself up such that only the hands are touching the ground. One hovers briefly and then, without the feet touching the mat, begins to exhale and (magically, it seems) slowly swings one's chest forward and hips and legs backward at the same time, landing in chaturanga dandasana (low plank pose).

This posture is followed by urdhva mukha shvanasana (upward-facing dog pose; see figure 5.1), adho mukha shvanasana (downward-facing dog pose), and then, in a single controlled movement, the jump-through – a slow forward jump in which the whole lower body is moved through one's arms such that one lands softly in dandasana (staff pose; see figure 5.2). During the jump-back and jump-through, the body appears to float.

This sequence of moves – sometimes referred to by the shorthand term "vinyasa" – has been part of modern postural yoga for decades, with photographs and film footage of Tirumalai Krishnamacharya, Pattabhi Jois, and B.K.S. Iyengar demonstrating their mastery of this elegant transition. It is also ubiquitous in social media and found in several styles of yoga (e.g., power, Jivamukti, and vinyasa). It has a special place in Jois's asana series, where it occurs dozens of times. This transition is quite difficult to do smoothly and is valued because it creates tapas (heat), builds strength, and truth be told, impresses others.

"Do it again," said Jamie, a thirty-two-year-old advanced teacher, in a markedly unimpressed voice.

I looked up from dandasana. "Sorry, what?"

"Do it again," he said as he leaned over to help someone with karnapidasana (ear press pose; see figure 5.3) a few mats away.

"Do I have to?" I asked with a bit of a whine in my voice, acutely aware that the room was entirely silent except for the measured breathing of other students.

Jamie cocked his head quickly and looked at me as though I had just spoken Danish. "Excuse me?"

"Right. Joking. Okay, here," I whispered. Then I breathed in and performed the vinyasa as I exhaled. Looking up, I noticed that he had moved to the front of the room.

In a flat, clear voice, he said, "We all see you can do it with your arms, but that's not the point. The core is the point, so why are you relying on your

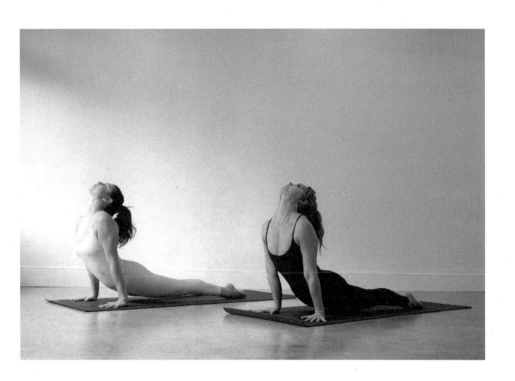

Figure 5.1
Urdhva mukha shvanasana (upward-facing dog pose)

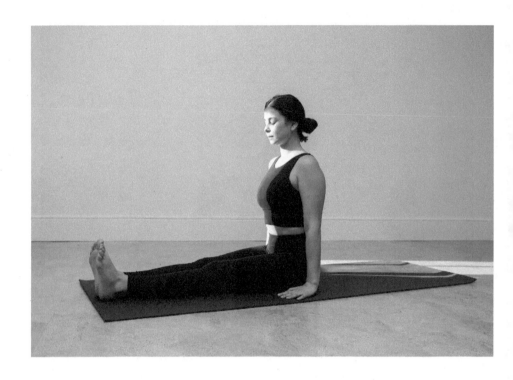

Figure 5.2
Dandasana (staff pose)

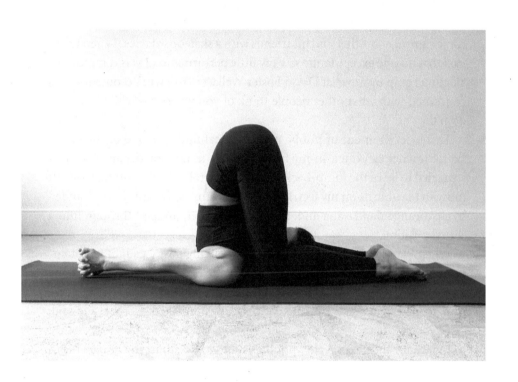

Figure 5.3
Karnapidasana (ear press pose)

arms? Do it again." He watched as I repeated the move. "Again." I did it once more. "Okay, that's better."

This intervention stung not mainly because of his imperative tone and the fact that I would need to repeat this challenging transition. It was, instead, the "We all see you can …" part that chafed a little because, indeed, he had noticed that I had wanted him and everyone else to see my vinyasa. I had known him for perhaps twenty-five minutes, but Jamie saw me (correctly, I have to say) as a proud six-year-old who wanted to impress his cooler, stronger brother and his friends with a skateboard trick. When I realized that no one except Jamie saw my little performance, I was reminded of a famous quip by novelist David Foster Wallace: "You will become way less concerned with what other people think of you when you realize how seldom they do."[12]

This brief moment of public psychological nudity is one of the gifts a skilful teacher can offer. In my first two years in my practice in Victoria, I struggled to learn the jump-back. After innumerable sweaty failures had left me with mat-burns on my feet, I finally swung my body through and landed in chaturanga dandasana and, a few breaths later, jumped through into a seated position.

When I landed, my teacher, Annie, was walking past. I caught her attention. "Did you see that?" I asked, gleefully. She had noticed and was happy that I had crossed a certain threshold. She also saw the danger in my question, so instead of answering me, she playfully mimicked my tone, and said, "Did you see that?"

In fact, for the next several months as she would adjust me or pass me in the foyer, she would occasionally whisper, "Did you see that?"

But back to Manhattan. When Jamie engaged me in this brusque manner in front of a group of strangers, I was embarrassed, but I smiled because I had a keen sense of how odd it is to find myself in situations where teachers (many of whom I barely know) treat me in ways that I would never accept from friends, family members, neighbours, strangers, or even bosses.[13]

What does this quite time-and-place-specific style of interaction tell us? In the older lineages – such as those linked to the father of modern postural yoga, Krishnamacharya – one finds oneself in the presence of the ancient guru-shishya (student) model, which is central to Indic teachings and communities. Alicia, a senior Iyengar teacher we met in New York, observed,

So in the guru[-shishya] model, if you're willing to give yourself over, and you believe this guru, this teacher, knows everything I need, and you just give yourself, then you feel safe. Because you've given over, you're trusting the method, you're trusting the teacher and you can go with that. And I think to a certain extent you do have a better yoga experience if you're not fighting the yoga. I mean, you have to be open to it to a certain extent. But then I think that there's a certain level of safety that comes when the student trusts you. Not because you are all knowing but because there's some sense of compassion.

The guru-shishya model, even if especially evident in the relatively India-oriented systems (certainly Iyengar, Ashtanga, Kripalu, Sivananda, Bikram, and Dharma Mittra), is not unique to yoga settings, of course; it is an integral part of Asian cultures and histories.

Here, a quick digression into popular culture history might illustrate what I mean. The 1984 film *The Karate Kid* was a massive hit in its time and has lived on in popular culture through the 2010 remake with Jackie Chan and Jayden Smith, through its 2018 reboot as the Netflix series *Cobra Kai*, and through memes such as "wax on, wax off." A significant moment in the movie was the tension between the young American boy Daniel LaRusso (Ralph Macchio) and the inscrutable Japanese gardener-cum-sensei Mr Miyagi (Pat Morita). When LaRusso asks Miyagi to teach him martial arts, LaRusso is asked to paint the fence and wash the car instead of being trained to fight. This regimen infuriates LaRusso, but more than that, it demonstrates a common Asian teacher-student, or guru-shishya, power structure.

Eventually, of course, the wisdom animating this power structure is revealed when LaRusso finds that hours of tedious fence painting and car cleaning ("wax on, wax off!") have given him the physical strength and balance that he needs to challenge a bully (and to attract a girl, of course).

At one point, Miyagi says to LaRusso, "[We] must make sacred pact. I promise [to] teach karate. That [is] my part. You promise [to] learn. I say, you do. No question. That [is] your part. Deal?"

Many students feel supported and respected in these relationships – especially when, to use Alicia's term, they are based on compassion (as they clearly are in *The Karate Kid*). For my part, I accept – indeed, welcome – Ashtanga and Iyengar teachers' imperious tone because I know that it demonstrates both a site- and time-limited expression of tenderness and interest in me and my practice.

Indeed, as a straight, male, white-passing, full professor with plenty of social capital, I was perhaps masochistically drawn to the opportunity to feel utterly incompetent and then, after a decade of daily practice with advanced teachers, to feel reasonably competent. The point is that guru-shishya relationships are far removed from the egalitarian, self-esteem-validating ethos that is increasingly indicative of work, teaching, and social spaces in Canada and the United States. My academic peers would certainly find it strange to watch me return every day to spaces where, to paraphrase Mr. Miyagi, *they say, and I do – no question.*

Thanks to a general atmosphere of reverence around the founders, teachings, and often family members of the founders (in the case of Ashtanga and Iyengar, for example), new students in lineage-based sites quickly learn the appropriate habitus (or norms or attitudes) of the community and the centrality of the hierarchical teacher-student power structure. Nonetheless, for visitors to these sites, it is alarming to see a teacher use such an imperative tone – "Do it *again*, Mallory. No, I said your *right* hip. Your. Right. Hip" – which would be obnoxious outside of the studio given that Mallory is a vice-president of a Fortune 500 company and that the teacher is a barista when she is not teaching yoga.

I do not want to overstate the difference between the relational approaches within and outside of studios: interactions range from terse to transactional to tender. Nonetheless, I do think that in many cases, the differences between the relational patterns would be quite noticeable (and perhaps irritating) to newcomers. Whenever I bring a friend or a student to my shala I prepare them for the ethos and authority structure that they are about to enter because they reflect an Indian approach to teacher-student relations that some Westerners might find off-putting.

Central to the guru-shishya model is the claim or assumption that the South Asian founders or lineage holders – Iyengar, Jois, Swami Sivananda, Amrit Desai, Kausthub Desikachar, Bikram Choudhury, and all the rest – have a special relationship not just to Patanjali's third limb of yoga (i.e., asana) but to the other seven limbs as well. According to the lore built into most traditions, the founders or gurus in question do not just intellectually understand the full power of yoga's promises but have also realized these powers. Moreover, one's local North American teacher often has some kind of special relationship with the Indian lineage holder since usually they have met the founder or his heirs and have spent time working with them in Pune, Mysore, Rishikesh, Goa, or any number of workshop or training sites around the world. Through these direct or indirect personal connections, teachers in Florida, Manitoba, Idaho, or Quebec are imagined to have had access to the mystery and majesty of yoga's authentic and original Indian form.

The often rough guru-shishya relational style is not merely an echo of timeless ancient patterns but also a reflection of very specific experiences of the founders of modern postural yoga. Consider, for example, B.K.S. Iyengar's visit to the United Kingdom in 1954. Although dedicated contemporary practitioners may be teased by friends and neighbours, Indian teachers such as Iyengar often had a much more difficult time being taken seriously in the initial decades of yoga's expansion in the West. In his final interview in 2014, he shared a memory that reveals just how much his personal difficulties shaped the yoga that he taught for decades.

The British never allowed me even to have tea [i.e., dinner] with other people. I was segregated because I was an Indian; I was a slave. I was eating only bread and coffee because there were no vegetables even available. They used to say, "This grass-eater has so much strength" ... I accepted all these things [i.e., indignities]. Do people know that? They were calling me a slave. So I had in my mind that I will be a slave driver to these slave drivers. Outside I did not explain [that] I will one day treat you like that. But I made them. Now, in the early books they would ask, "What does B.K.S. stand for?" Beating, kicking, and shouting. Now today the same people say it [stands] for beauty, knowledge, and serenity ... Now you can imagine what transformation has taken place from beating to beauty.[14]

My stomach tightened when I realized that Iyengar's story echoes those I heard from my father and others from the Indian and Caribbean diasporas who moved to Britain or Canada in the 1960s, expecting to be welcomed. There, they encountered among their new neighbours the firm conviction that subaltern brown people ought to be grateful that their ancestors were brought into the beneficent orbit of British civilization. The indignities that Iyengar experienced in his early days in the West resulted in the legendary ferocity of his teaching and left a mark on other teachers that we can still see even sixty years after this experience.

The disgrace was not endured only by Iyengar. Millions of other South Asians – and South Asians in the colonial diaspora, like my family – resented their secondary status for centuries. Their resistance was expressed in various ways and culminated in the 1947 British exit from India and in the disastrous partition of India and Pakistan, the latter being a trauma from which the region has yet to heal. The formal dissent against centuries of British rule has been the subject of a massive scholarly and journalistic literature.

Opposition took many forms. When Krishnamacharya was asked by the raja of Mysore to teach yoga to the boys of the palace, he combined extant asana traditions with the "physical culture" of the British military tradition and the gymnastics of Scandinavian exercise manuals.[15] It is easy to forget that many of the asanas that Krishnamacharya taught Iyengar and Jois, which are now staples of North American yoga communities, were practised by very few people throughout the history of South Asia.

Krishnamacharya's asanas – some new, some old, and some revised but all systematized and newly bound together by his vinyasa system, which married breath and movement – were initially meant not only to strengthen the boys of the palace and others who joined the group but also, one may speculate, to challenge the British stereotype of the effete, listless, servile Indian man.[16] Krishnamacharya's demanding, graceful, muscular yoga helped to empower, and even to liberate, the permanently marginal object of colonial disdain: the slave, to use Iyengar's term.

With the help of yogic practices birthed on Indian soil but fortified and "modernized" through aspects of European physical culture, the practitioners who (knowingly or not) followed the lead of Krishnamacharya participated in the nationalist movement. The interactions that took place between the West and India – both when Indians such as Jois and Iyengar came to the West to teach and when Westerners went to India to learn – need to be understood against the backdrop of India's emancipation efforts and of the tendency among Westerners to see India as a bastion of spiritual wisdom and mystery that they felt could not be found in their home societies.[17]

Now, many decades later, relatively orthodox – or actually "orthoprax" since the emphasis is on correct practice rather than on belief – Ashtanga and Iyengar teachers who employ the brusque teaching methods of their Indian lineage founders have complicated feelings about how they were taught by the twentieth-century masters. Alicia, a senior Iyengar teacher, noted,

> I don't need to shout at my students and humiliate my students, which has happened and which I have witnessed [in the past, from Indian teachers such as Iyengar] ... You know, if I took my current self back fifteen or ten years ago, I wouldn't be able to stay in those [classes]. Like I think I would walk out, whereas at the time I was just *in it*, and I wasn't the one getting yelled at ... It is different now, too, that because Iyengar is gone ... I can't shout at my students like that. Was it effective when he taught? I enjoyed some of what he did, but I would never teach that way to my students.[18]

Many other teachers continue to pass along to their students the same fierce ethos that they learned from the masters, often unaware that this style was informed to a large extent by colonial humiliation. Sometimes this model of teaching is appreciated by these students (like me), who perhaps counterintuitively value the opportunity to surrender some agency in pursuit of healing and insight. I would stridently protest the rough treatment that I sometimes experience in a studio if it occurred anywhere else – but the shala is not like anywhere else. In these spaces, and only there, people are granted a licence to treat – to touch, to address, to tease, to support – others in ways that they would never consider outside of this anti-world.

It is both poignant and amusing to see the thread connecting the *Yoga Sutras*, my likely Brahmin ancestors, the humiliation of millions of Indians in (and after) the British Empire, and a part-time Iyengar teacher and full-time neurologist with chunky black glasses who admonishes me, "I've told you three times already – turn your left foot *in*." This brilliant teacher is not aware that my mind is connecting histories – from ancient India to 1947 India to 1954 Britain to 1960 Canada to a mat in contemporary Indianapolis – so she does not understand why I smile in response to her sometimes tyrannical techniques.

Two Cracks in the Veneer

Even if one understands postural yoga in North America as increasingly North American,[19] it is impossible to understand this phenomenon without reflecting on the well-burnished ideas of India, Indians, and Indianness. I think of India as a load-bearing wall in the deep infrastructure of almost all yoga communities: you do not usually see it, but without it, the integrity of the whole building is severely compromised. This foundation was jeopardized by two recent cultural movements.

Yogaland's #MeToo Moment

I think that it is fair to say that many North Americans assume that the lives of women over the past five or six decades have improved meaningfully, with victories around equal pay, access to reproductive health services, parental rights, divorce and spousal abuse legislation, political representation, and increased access to once exclusively male professions, such as medicine, law, engineering, and military service. One might well question whether the changes in women's civil and human rights are substantive and complete or merely distractions from the control exerted by pernicious ideologies (especially neoliberalism). I mention the consensus that exists in the political and public stories around women's gradually improved latitude just to set the stage.

Regardless of how one might characterize the situation of contemporary women, very few men or women were fully prepared for the massive public articulation of pain that we saw in 2017. In 2006, Tarana Burke started the Me Too movement to create a context in which women could share experiences of sexual violence. Now, however, when people use the phrase, they usually have in mind the #MeToo phenomenon, which began when the American actor Alissa Milano attached a hashtag to the slogan in a 2017 tweet describing her own abuse. She invited other women to include this slogan in their social media posts if they, too, had been victims. Her suggestion lit up social media for the next two or three years.

The media focused on the more grotesque characters in this controversy, such as Harvey Weinstein and Bill Cosby, but there was an unquenchable thirst for other names and backstories. We saw the fall of other high-profile figures such as Kevin Spacey, Matt Lauer, Al Franken, Bill Hybels, Jian Ghomeshi, Louis C.K., and Charlie Rose. The unethical behaviour of many thousands of others, from all walks of life, has been exposed in the process, and workplaces have rushed either to strengthen or to create sexual violence prevention protocols. The range of accusations is very wide, from violent rape to unwanted advances to inappropriate teasing and everything in between. The victims have almost exclusively been women and girls, although on occasion (as in the Spacey case), boys or men were involved. Milano's 2017 tweet vastly expanded the #MeToo movement, which gained so much traction that it is now both a specific phenomenon and a broad movement for justice and truth telling that encompasses events that happened even before the hashtag began to circulate.[20]

The list of men accused or guilty of misconduct is long, and no sphere of society was untouched. When priests, politicians, teachers, and coaches were identified, there were pre-existing media tropes that could be used to describe perpetrators and victims. When so many previously beloved celebrities (such as Cosby, Rose, Ghomeshi, and Spacey) were named and when vast numbers of women came forward on social media to accuse so many others or even just to post a simple #MeToo with no additional context, the epidemic nature of these experiences shocked many of us. Some predictably said that they knew all along that such misconduct was pervasive, but it was still hard not to be overwhelmed by the sheer scale of the claims.

The movement also cut like a scythe through yogaland and impacted virtually every lineage and style. There were certainly scandals that predated 2017, but few anticipated just how pervasive the problem was until #MeToo discussions arrived in studios. A full list of those credibly accused would be very long. Indeed, many of the often whispered accusations concerning local teachers resulted in these teachers simply withdrawing from teaching duties (or, of course, moving to other studios or styles), so they never received much media attention. Here is an abbreviated list of the high-profile figures, with their practices or lineages and the approximate date of the scandal's public emergence given in parentheses:

- Muktananda Paramahamsa (Siddha – 1980s)
- Swami Nithyananda (Siddha – 1985)
- Satchidananda Saraswati (Integral – 1991)

- Amrit Desai (Kripalu – 1994)
- Swami Rama (Yoga Nidra – 1997)
- Rodney Yee (Iyengar, etc. – 2002)
- Kausthub Desikachar, grandson of Krishnamacharya (Viniyoga – 2012)
- John Friend (Anusara – 2012)
- David Life (Jivamukti – 2016)
- Manouso Manos (Iyengar – 2018)
- Pattabhi Jois (Ashtanga – 2017)
- Vishnudevananda Saraswati (Sivananda – 2019)
- Bikram Choudhury (Bikram – 2019)
- Yogi Bhajan (Kundalini – 2019)[21]

This incomplete list mentions those teachers with significant followings who were often treated as gurus and who either were Indians themselves or relied on their real or putative attachment to India or Indian gurus.[22] As I noted, although some of these revelations pre-date #MeToo, the movement brought fresh attention to past widespread allegations of misconduct.

Obviously, this book is not the place for a complete account of the misdeeds, media responses, legal remedies, or current state of these cases.[23] Nor is this context appropriate for a discussion of the ways that communities responded to these scandals and traumas. I should just note that many studio owners responded to these scandals by producing statements or codes of conduct that they put on their websites or posted in their common spaces. The Yoga Alliance, the largest and most influential professional association in the yoga industry, published quite a comprehensive statement on its website in 2020.[24] Also, "consent cards" – small plasticized cards with, for example, "yes, please" on one side and "no, thanks" on the other – were available in many communities. One could place these cards beside one's mat to indicate whether physical contact was welcome. In the spaces where I practised during #MeToo, these cards were available, and they continue to be in use today, although after a few months they were very rarely used because, I assume, the teachers came to understand which students welcomed which kind of interaction.

To illustrate the nature and impact of the #MeToo movement in yogaland, it is useful to offer very brief outlines of three prominent sexual misconduct scandals.[25]

Some of the worst stories swirl around Bikram Choudhury, whose hot yoga community was rocked by the 2014 *Vanity Fair* article "Bikram Feels the Heat," which brought into the open rumours that many of his earliest students (several of whom I met during fieldwork in Los Angeles) already knew to be true.[26] As Renée Marie Schettler notes, "In all, seven women – six of them former Bikram yoga students – filed civil lawsuits against Choudhury for sexual assault, harassment, creating a hostile work environment, wrongful termination, or rape. The Los Angeles District Attorney's Office has not chosen to pursue criminal charges against Choudhury."[27]

His legal woes culminated in 2016 with penalties of over US$7 million ordered by a Los Angeles Superior Court. Bikram fled the United States to escape this decision and potential future civil and criminal charges. His troubles were massively amplified by the scathing documentary *Bikram: Yogi, Guru, Predator* (2019), launched at the peak of yoga's #MeToo movement.[28] Although it is an understatement to say that Bikram is not portrayed sympathetically, this graphic exposé of his narcissism, mendacity, misconduct, and overall creepiness – with plenty of footage of him in his famous black Speedo sitting on an air-conditioned platform while his students sweltered – did not destroy his teaching career. Indeed, he continues to teach his eponymous sequence and offer teacher trainings outside of the United States.[29]

In my interviews, quite a few people explained that Bikram had been their gateway into yoga. After his scandalous behaviour became the stuff of tabloids, talk shows, and legal history, his students faced a difficult dilemma. A handful of Bikram studios remain in North America, but the vast majority of them have dropped his name. In the wake of the legal and public relations fiasco that Bikram faced, Moksha Yoga (later, Modo), among other new companies, arose and continued to offer hot yoga classes. Some studios have kept many of the postures that he sought to trademark and, in fact, continue to offer some version of Bikram's sequence of twenty-six postures and two breathing exercises. These studios have also kept heating their spaces to about 40 degrees Celsius (105 degrees Fahrenheit) at about 40 per cent humidity.

What drew people to an environment that seems so oppressive to others, and what kept them there? None of the former students I met mounted a defence of Bikram as such, but they were also not reluctant to try to bring me into the world that he had built. In fact, many referred to the practice as profoundly life-altering. For example, Deepa, a seasoned Los Angeles teacher of South Asian descent (no longer exclusively teaching in heated rooms), described her first class with Bikram and explained its impact on her life:

> After the fifth pose, you get a little break, water break. You take the water break, and I leave, and I'm like, "My God, this is disgusting. I hate it. A hundred degrees. It's like a hundred people in here. What is this? This is like nuts." He came out [to the lobby, where I was taking a break], and he's like, "I guarantee by the end of the class [you will change your mind]. And I just want to make sure that we at least try." So I come back in, I get back in. It's in front of a mirror. And I'm in the front row, and all of a sudden something just happens for me in that mirror ... There's a lot of answers and a lot of questions and a download [of insight or wisdom] that can happen. And so this was starting to happen for me in the mirror in this class. And by the end of the class, it was just, I was sold. I was like, "Oh my God, this is life-changing." He asked if he could train me as a teacher and [said] that he was putting his first teacher-training group together. And I said, yes. I spent $10,000 to be in this training for six months, six days a week, nine in the morning to nine at night. And it changed my, just completely changed my life.

Although this was not part of Deepa's story, many others highlighted the effect that hot yoga has had on their mental health and spiritual quests. Bella, a studio owner in Los Angeles, spoke of "waking up":

> And I went [into the room], and it was packed! It was like, "This dark room with like, half naked bodies." And I was like, "Oh my gosh, what is this?" And I just fell in love right away ... And one day, I was just like, "This is changing me." I'm like, "I'm waking up." Like I was really, felt like I was waking up. And, and I think, you know, I knew what it was. I knew it was that, that I was in such a stressful time in my life. I was working so many hours. I was at this [corporate job] and like trying to strive in this man's world and like trying to keep up and like, and I wasn't happy. And so it was like slowing me down – the two-minute

shavasana [corpse pose] changed my life, you know? I can actually just like breathe. And then lay down and like be in my skin and my bones and not try to be something that I'm not.

Cindy, a former hot yoga student and now a teacher of several different yoga types in Los Angeles, observed,

One day, one of my friends came up to me, and she was like, "Come take a yoga class." And I was like, "Hmm, no, absolutely not. That's not my jam." And she was like, "No, please come take a yoga class." And I was like, "Okay, you know what? Sure, I'll try this. Why not?" And I took a heated Bikram class. That was my first class ever. I was wearing long leggings, a cotton T-shirt. It was brutal. But when I walked out, I was like, "Wow, I feel amazing." And at the time, I was severely depressed, and it just made me feel a little less depressed. And so I started practising all the time. And shortly after that, I got crazy into it and was taking three heated classes a day, seven days a week.

Kadisha, an African American teacher in Los Angeles, noted that when she took Bikram's classes in 2012, she initially thought, "I couldn't hardly think about anything except the heat and being in that room. And I was like, 'Okay, I like this. It's a little aggressive, but I like this.'" Similarly, Pamela, a Canadian colleague of mine who practised Bikram yoga for many years, explained, "I have a lot of anxiety issues, but when I'm in that space, all I can think about is survival. That really focuses the mind. Also, just being around people who are all suffering in the same way – well, it creates a sense of community pretty fast."

Other practitioners, however, remember Bikram and the practice differently. Even Deepa noted, "Bikram himself is crazy, and he's gotten crazier and crazier and crazier … I found him to be humorous. I didn't find it offensive. Some people would find it offensive, you know, I mean, [but] there's a lot of people getting offended over a lot of things today." Laura, now a senior teacher in Los Angeles, said,

The first time I practised yoga was in the [late] seventies with Bikram, and I hated it. There was a woman [in class] that said something about

God, you know, which is interesting. And he got very upset with her. And, you know, he's just this little guy. And he picked her up, and he literally threw her out of the class. And at that time, this is like 1973, and he pulled $20 out of the cash register and threw it at her. And he told her to never come back again. And I thought, "I hate yoga. I am never going to do this again."

Laura did eventually find another home, within the Ashtanga system, which is the site of the second scandal that I would like to sketch briefly.

By way of an entry into this story, let me share a vignette from my 2023 Ashtanga vinyasa teacher training. As one of our assignments, we watched the documentary *Mysore Magic: Yoga at the Source* (2012) by R. Alexander Medin. The film introduces prospective participants to the unique physical, social, and spiritual features of both Mysore in southern India and its main Ashtanga shala. One of the students interviewed by Medin comments, "[Mysore is] this strangely undefinable thing that you have to just come and experience." To underline her claim about the uniqueness of the city and the shala, another student says, "It's impossible to taste the sweetness of sugar without putting it in your mouth." By way of an explanation for why Mysore loomed so large in his mind, a third practitioner said, "I always associated yogis with superheroes."[30]

As I noted earlier, the southern Indian city of Mysore is the symbolic heart of the Ashtanga world. It is where Krishnamacharya taught the boys of the palace, and it is where he worked with Iyengar and Jois, the leaders of the two main lineage systems in North America that have massively influenced other forms of postural yoga throughout the world.

Pattabhi Jois, the leader of the Ashtanga lineage, had died three years before *Mysore Magic* was made, but his spirit suffuses the film. He is mentioned lovingly many times, and his image is shown on the walls of the shala and other spaces featured in the film. The most famous of the Westerners interviewed is the American yoga superstar Kino MacGregor. Everyone in the film needed to apply formally to Jois's grandson Sharath Jois, the current lineage holder, for permission to spend time (usually several months each visit) in Mysore working on asana practice, learning philosophy, chanting, and otherwise deepening their practice.

The film shifts smoothly from interviews with articulate practitioners to scenes of the surrounding cityscape – with colourful markets, coconut stands, roads, temples, palaces, and commercial buildings – to the inside of what was then the main practice room in Mysore. In this space, viewers not only see Mysore-style practice, in which students work on the Ashtanga sequence and are assisted by teachers walking around the room, but also see a class in which Sharath Jois leads a group through an advanced series of postures.

Practitioners in the video share thoughtful stories about the power of the practice and the lineage in their healing, self-understanding, and relationships with others. I do not want to cast aspersions on the ways that they talk about the value of their practice, which resonate in some ways with what I characterized in this book's introduction as my own "Amazing Grace" conversion story. I mention this film simply because, although officially it concerns and promotes the Ashtanga system and the Mysore shala, it is also a hagiography – literally a saint-writing exercise, or to use a concept that I have noted in this book, an authorizing and discourse-generating exercise. Through the film, the deceased guru Pattabhi Jois and his grandson the paramaguru Sharath Jois together embody, authenticate, and safeguard the magic of Mysore.[31]

Regardless of the religious, spiritual, or social tradition in which such hagiographical exercises take place, they are always interesting cases to consider, especially since the generators of these saint stories rely on common techniques to convey their message. In 2012, Jois's name was not yet synonymous with the scandals that would grip the yoga world less than a decade later. The film was – to return to the Yeats poem at the beginning of this chapter – a ceremony of innocence, and with the value of hindsight, it is somewhat poignant to watch the film now that we have a more complete sense of the shortcomings of the lineage founder.

The end of this ceremony of innocence came in November 2017 when a very advanced teacher, Karen Rain, announced on Facebook that "Pattabhi Jois sexually assaulted me regularly during his yoga *asana* 'adjustments.'" Rain's post was inspired by "Yoga Girl" Rachel Brathen's pleas for people in the global yoga community to contribute to the #MeToo conversation. In 2018, Rain published a longer blog post with the title "Yoga Guru Pattabhi

Jois Sexually Assaulted Me for Years." Many community members were shocked both by her story and by the photographs of adjustments that she felt were sexual and problematic. She provided a rationale for these pictures: "I consented to publishing these images in part because they are evidence of Pattabhi Jois abusing me, but also because he should be remembered this way: He was not just the smiling guru on the yoga altar. He was also a man who violated women in full view of other people. I want the photos to be a call for everyone to examine whether they are dismissing or overlooking sexual abuse in any way."[32]

Other practitioners came forward to confirm that they, too, had observed or experienced similar problematic adjustments or straightforward misconduct.[33] In the wake of these revelations, Sharath Jois issued a response that many in the community felt was too little or too late, as it came well over a year after Rain's 2017 brief announcement and over two months after her longer 2018 post.[34] There were many responses to the guarded tone of the official statement by the junior Jois, but suffice it to say that many people (myself included) were unsatisfied.

Interestingly, several senior teachers I met sought to place Pattabhi Jois's behaviour within the context of his sheltered life. Laura, in California, said, "You have to bear in mind that he was a small-town Brahmin, and quite conservative. And then, all of a sudden in the 1970s and 1980s he was surrounded almost every day with super confident Western women maybe between twenty and thirty, wearing almost no clothes. He would never have seen women like this. I mean, it's like if you put a kid on a chair and put a bunch of lollipops in front of him and then say, 'Don't lick those.' Eventually he will lick them."

I appreciate Laura's effort to situate Jois within his personal and cultural context, even though her account tends to infantilize him and perhaps by extension other Indian men – who, like unsophisticated boys, should not be expected to control their impulses, I suppose. I imagine that this lollipop analogy might, for some (yet, to be clear, not for me), excuse his behaviour. But even if one accepts that he might have been initially disoriented by the presence of so many minimally clad women from around the world who wanted to learn from and to be adjusted by him, the novelty of this initial exposure does not seem like a compelling explanation for behaviour that lasted for many years.[35]

The situation is complicated, of course. A senior teacher in the United States noted that she had studied with Jois for years and had neither seen nor experienced anything resembling the claims made by others. Phoebe's story was one of the unique gifts uncovered by our use of the ethnographic method, which exposes you to people's real lives in a way that surveys, questionnaires, and dispassionate theorizing rarely do. She said,

> I trust people's experience, and I don't want to invalidate that. But the thing I came to is that I also don't want to invalidate my own. And that wasn't my experience. And in fact, [Jois's adjustments were] the most healing thing in my life and helped me heal from other places where I did feel violated. And so, yeah *[pause]*, I also know most of the people who have come forward, and most of them have a pretty intense history of trauma. And so, again, not to invalidate it, but just to say there might be certain things that triggered it … I spent a couple years thinking [about how to respond to these claims], but it's like, for me, [to join the condemnation of Jois] takes away from my experience, and that's not fair.

During fieldwork in the United States I met a major figure in the Ashtanga scene who said that after the #MeToo revelations, she ultimately concluded that the elder Jois was an excellent asana teacher but not a guru. This interpretation certainly stands in contrast with the perspective of a few other teachers I met from the same lineage, who still have photos of Jois on altars in their shalas, but the more skeptical American in question is perhaps established enough that she no longer needs the imprimatur (or official approval) provided by close affiliation with Mysore and the Jois family.

I was attracted to Ashtanga not by its once revered founder or by his grandson, the so-called paramaguru Sharath Jois, but by my local teachers and by the physical repair that the practice allowed. So there was very little at stake for me when the Jois scandal broke. Nonetheless, I did wonder whether the storm of controversy around these issues might end the Ashtanga community, just as the controversies around yoga teacher John Friend's sexual misconduct had ostensibly ended the Anusara brand.[36] When I brought the issue up with Ashtangis at studios in 2022 and 2023, some did offer anguished reflections, but many clearly needed to search their memories for specific details of the scandal so that they could respond.

There are certainly people practising now – even long-term students and teachers with whom I practise – who either did not pay attention to the controversies when they arose or felt that the controversies were not relevant to their own practice. Perhaps people were able to move on because when the claims about his misconduct entered the public arena in 2017, the attention devoted to new high-profile people named every week during the #MeToo movement may have diluted the energy one could give to Jois, who had died in 2009.

I came late to this accident scene. I did not begin my own practice in 2013 with any interest in lineages of any kind (and I remain indifferent to them now). The lineage founder – I do not think that I even heard the Jois name for several weeks – had died years before I started my practice, and the grandson was 13,000 kilometres away. My arthritis was so distressing and I had so much to learn from Jack and Annie that the fact that they were both emotionally and practically attached to the authority and magic of the Mysore tradition was not very relevant for me. Although I have Indian roots, have visited India, and am generally curious about all religious communities, I was in this case narrowly interested in effective physiotherapy and thought that I might also benefit from the stress management that people often said yoga could deliver.

The scandal finally became a problem when Rain and others came forward, at which point I felt that I needed to take some kind of position on the abuses that they had catalogued with such detail. My stance in the conversation was predictable and not terribly innovative. In short: the conduct of yoga teachers named during #MeToo, including Jois, was reprehensible and inexcusable. The current leaders owe the victims an unequivocal apology and perhaps other kinds of compensation. This crisis was an opportunity for all yoga communities to assess their formal and informal norms, including when and how to touch students and what kind of intimacies would be permitted between teachers and students outside of studios. My position on the abuse reflects my suspicion – not uncommon among colleagues in my field – of all spiritualized authority structures that direct aspirants through a narrow gate.

I do not argue with fellow practitioners who do not embrace my position. The stakes are much lower for me than for other practitioners who have had life-changing experiences in Mysore, after all. I have not built my identity, my practice, or my peer group around any real or imagined relationship with the magic of Mysore. As well, I am not trying to sustain a community that since the 1980s has been oriented toward Mysore in much the same way that mosques around the world are oriented toward Mecca. My position might be different if, like Phoebe, I had experienced the deep and singular healing that she experienced with Pattabhi Jois and, further, if my position in the yoga economy was contingent on an unofficial affiliation with a particular family or an official Mysore-dependent "authorization" or "certification" to teach.[37]

The third and final story to consider concerns the Sivananda community, founded by Swami Sivananda (d. 1963), and continued by his successor, Swami Vishnudevananda (d. 1993).[38] At the height of #MeToo, Vishnudevananda's assistant, Julie Salter, revealed in a Facebook post that she had endured many years of sexual mistreatment at his hands. Thanks to Salter's 2019 post, a large amount of corroborating evidence was subsequently amassed against Vishnudevananda.[39]

When I visited one of the main Sivananda spaces in North America, I noticed that Vishnudevananda's books continued to be sold and that his images were featured prominently on the walls throughout the building. Indeed, in at least one of the practice rooms that I visited during a tour, his image was surrounded with a garland.

It is a standard operating procedure in ethnographies to ask interview subjects to read and sign a detailed consent form, which includes information about the project, their role in it, and their ability to withdraw at any time. I am never sure how closely people read these forms. Still, I try to be very delicate when raising allegations of sexual misconduct within communities that have lived through – or are still living through – the legal, moral, and public strife that these controversies create. One never really knows how people will respond even to the most cautious, open-ended questions. In this interview, however, it became immediately apparent how the conversation would unfold.

When I asked a senior practitioner about the place of honour that Vishnudevananda continued to have within the community's buildings, libraries, and public-facing digital spaces, even after Salter's claims, he balked. It looked to me like he was trying to decide between fight or flight. He chose the former.

He growled, "So are you trying to tell me that sexual abuse doesn't happen in companies? So are you going to close down Amazon and other companies?"

I was confused by this analogy, but I assume that he meant that in any large group and even in corporations that many consider to be integral to our societies, there will always be bad people and undesirable behaviour. I tried to lighten the mood of the interview by replying to his question about Amazon with a joke that, "Well, [closing down Amazon] might be a good idea for many other reasons." Frankly, his mood was not lightened, and I suddenly felt a sense of dread as he sat back in his chair, furrowed his brow, and continued.

"I'm just saying, are you going to throw out the baby with the bathwater? Because the bathwater is dirty, are you going to throw the baby out with it?"

My heart raced. I tried to assure him that I was neither a journalist nor a lawyer and was not looking to embarrass or chastise him; nor was I there to uncover new details about the scandal itself. I reiterated the key questions of my project, all of which were outlined on the consent form. I explained that although the project was certainly not focused on sexual abuse controversies, the response of communities to allegations in almost all yoga communities nonetheless provided insights into the ways that groups might adjust to changing public norms, reimagine themselves in light of crises, and so forth.

In an effort to turn down the temperature in the interview, I noted that these problems had plagued the – that is, "my" – Ashtanga lineage too. I shared with him how some of my teachers and fellow students had responded to the news that Jois had been sexually inappropriate with some of his students. I indicated that members of the Ashtanga community had learned a great deal from these episodes about the inherent problems of the guru-shishya relationship and about changing ideas around sexual intimacy.

He took in my stories about the Ashtanga scandal but (understandably) seemed most concerned about the implications of the Salter allegations for his group and perhaps for himself. He was raised in South Asia and was in his late sixties, having spent many decades working as a volunteer (or "karma yogi") for the Sivananda community. Given other personal details that he shared about his life trajectory, I suspect that his material resources were li-

174

mited, which might explain why he was so defensive. He seemed caught in an unenviable position and somewhat stranded in his current role.

He continued his response. "Because then [if the swami's prominence is reduced and if the community declines], what is there left in classical yoga practice, and what are you going to learn? Who are you going to learn from? Who is going to teach it to you?"

This interview was, by a very wide margin, the most uncomfortable thirty-five minutes I have ever experienced since I began using this method in 1995. So many impressions and emotions collided in the discussion. I was certainly intellectually fascinated by the defence that he was mounting of the prominence of Vishnudevananda, but I also felt a deep impulse to escape. I resisted this urge, of course, and I am glad that I did since the experience revealed a great deal about the way that this community, or at least this person, responded to the crisis. It seemed to me that he was so used to talking with lawyers, communications consultants, and journalists that he could not quite accept that I was not trying to determine the veracity of either side's claims. Although in truth I had strong opinions about the matter, those are concerns to be taken up by others. In this case, I was just curious about how groups survive the tumult associated with these kinds of events.

The space between our chairs seemed to crackle with tension. I had a strong sense of what Patanjali meant by citta vritti (fluctuations of the mind). In other interviews with Ashtanga, Iyengar, Bikram, Kripalu, and Anusara practitioners, I raised the sexual misconduct scandals in their communities. In some cases – as with Laura's comment about lollipops – I bristled at what I heard, and people might have been defensive for a brief period. Without exception, however, they shared their opinions about the allegations and then responded to my underlying questions about the ramifications of the scandals and what the community learned from the events.

But in this case, the whole mood of the conversation darkened the moment that I introduced this issue, and a cloud hovered over the rest of the rather perfunctory discussion. I had arranged to take a class in their main practice space the next morning, but when I saw the garland around the framed picture, I felt nauseous. I might be wrong, but the age and layout of the building (which included living and practice spaces) suggested that the swami may have stayed there, perhaps with his assistant. After some soul-searching, I decided to cancel my registration for the class. Somehow being vulnerable, and perhaps touched, in that space seemed impossible.

When I came home, I told a friend about this unsettling experience. She said that she understood why I had decided not to practise in that studio the next day, but she also challenged me. "But you can practise in an Ashtanga setting in which there might still be a picture of Pattabhi Jois on the walls, right?"

She raised a good, and for me very uncomfortable, question. In response, I said that I would never have such a photograph in my own studio (if I were ever to open one) and that I would certainly raise this issue with the owner of any studio that I attended regularly. Fortunately, in the two shalas where I have spent most of my time, the teachers removed the photos as soon as the scandals emerged, so it was never an issue. However, I can tolerate being a guest in an Ashtanga shala with his photograph in it, and I do have friends who have his photo on their altars or who refer to Jois's famous insights when they teach. In my defence – and in a gesture that clearly reflects some magical thinking on my part – when I visit spaces in which his photo is still visible, I position my mat as far away from the picture as possible. This is a rather tepid response, I confess.

I have heard older practitioners who have met Jois say that his violations were less egregious than those of others, such as Bikram. But it is difficult, perhaps futile, to place yogaland's scandal-plagued leaders, including Jois, on a moral spectrum since I do not know the intimate details involved in these cases. I suppose that I feel some consolation in knowing that in almost all of the North American Ashtanga spaces that I have visited, these photos have been removed. But even this gesture is complicated. The disappearance of the images might reflect teachers' ethical responses to the scandals or a concern for marketing. But it might just as easily reflect the fact that more and more students who chant their gratitude to the long line of gurus at the beginning of most practices would not recognize either the name or the image of Pattabhi Jois.

There are many terms that galvanize the spiritual and temporal authority of a yogi in India, an Indian yogi abroad, or an India-indebted non-Indian yogi anywhere. Guru. Guruji. Parampara. Paramaguru. Boss. Yogacharya. Swami. Yogi. Siddha. Jivanmukta. Sri.[40]

When practitioners use these "honorifics," they might be doing little more than tipping their hat to accomplished or (since it often takes years to accomplish such things) mature practitioners. However, as the well-known Ashtanga teacher Eddie Stern reflected in an important 2019 *New Yorker Magazine* article, "I had this idea in me that the guru was supposed to be this all-encompassing everything ... I, along with other people, superimposed these mythologies on top of a human being [i.e., Jois] ... It was a misunderstanding of what the relationship was supposed to be."[41] This comment reveals not just one man's deep soul-searching with regard to his own lineage but also the crises in numerous yoga communities that have had to grapple with the painful revelations of the #MeToo era.

Most interesting is what he identifies as a very common tendency to assume that the guru has transcended normal human limitations and therefore deserves one's full and unquestioned obedience or veneration.[42] The debates over what it means to be or to follow a guru are long and complicated and best left to others to settle.[43] It is enough to note here that the matter is unresolved. Nonetheless, Talia, a member of Sadhguru's Isha yoga community, articulates a modest definition: "A guru is like a roadmap. It's not that you cannot reach the destination [on your own]. You can reach it, but you might wander for a very long time. [A guru] is someone who has walked the path. He knows the way. He's just guiding you and [showing you that] that's the shortest way. [Sadhguru sometimes] cracks a joke that GPS means 'guru positioning system.'"

Stern's insight, however, reminds us that it is not uncommon for gurus to do more than just orient you on a roadmap. Indeed, gurus often hint or claim, or have their followers hint or claim, that they have experienced advanced states of consciousness and that they – either they alone or they distinctively – can offer devotees access to these forms of awareness.

Achieving these states appears to be the driving force behind Patanjali's eight-limbed system. One of the reasons someone like Swami Vivekananda did not emphasize the first three limbs – yama, niyama, asana – was because he held, as did others, that their main role is to prepare people to pursue the more advanced goals of yoga, especially samadhi (meditative absorption) and kaivalya (solitude and liberation).

Consequently, it is not at all surprising that people might assume that gurus are not just talented at performing postures, breath work, or sense withdrawal but indeed are also masters of the whole yogic path. Given how explicit Patanjali's *Yoga Sutras* are about ethical behaviour – including the importance of the fourth yama, which is brahmacharya (literally "actions for the sake of Brahman"), usually defined as celibacy or conscientious sexual behaviour – it is no surprise that unethical sexual acts have created crises.

To put it very starkly: if so many of the gurus or the most trusted co-leaders in the gurus' lineages were unable to honour the very first yama – ahimsa (nonharming) – then how seriously can insiders take the guru or senior teachers when they talk about asana, not to mention samadhi? The matter is complicated by the fact that in many of these scandals, advanced practitioners were either (at best) compromised by their guru's charisma or (at worst) complicit in the victim blaming that occurred when allegations began to surface.[44]

Virtually all North American yoga communities are responding to sexual misconduct issues in one way or another, and it seems very unlikely that a single approach to dealing with these revelations will emerge. I do not have an (interesting) opinion on the best response. I am curious instead about the impact of the large cluster of scandals on the classic guru-shishya model. There is a lot riding on this impact since this model is at, or very near, the heart of the postural yoga tradition both in South Asia and in lineage-based communities in yogaland, including Ashtanga, Iyengar, the Self-Realization Fellowship, Sivananda, Dharma Mittra, Bikram, 3HO/Kundalini, Kripalu, and the Art of Living.

Some practitioners have found that only a definitive exit from their yoga community or postural yoga as such was an appropriate response to the reports, lawsuits, and trauma that we have seen over roughly the past decade.[45] But about five years after the peak of #MeToo, it seems that most people have found a way through.[46] The ground is still wet, but yogaland seems to have survived the flood.

Before I reflect on the way that #MeToo has destabilized yogaland, let us consider another crisis that might have a powerful impact on the often invisible authenticating power of India in North American yoga contexts.

Cultural Appropriation in Yogaland

During the past fifty years, there has emerged a fairly widespread awareness of the costs paid by subaltern people throughout history for the privileges enjoyed by citizens of Western liberal democracies. I do not want to argue that now we all know and act better. Obviously, racism, ethnocentrism, misogyny, and foreign meddling are not all in the past, as any honest reflection on the recent or current wars in Afghanistan, Iraq, Ukraine, and Israel-Palestine reveals. However, we need not look beyond North America for examples. The unfinished story of African American civil rights in the United States and the equally unresolved issue of Indigenous reconciliation in Canada provide plenty of reasons for remorse and national self-doubt.

Still, it can be said that in the public arena today, we hear fairly new discussions about performing in blackface, using the artistic styles associated with another culture, or using the image or name of Indigenous people to promote a sports team. These debates have their own histories, of course. In particular, Edward Said's groundbreaking *Orientalism* (1978) and then later Talal Asad's work[47] have helped many of us to appreciate the ways that one's notions of this or that exotic or threatening "other" reflect ethnocentric ideological biases that not coincidentally fit seamlessly with the political and economic interests of Western societies (or with the "civilization" that these societies comprise).

The responses that we have witnessed in yogaland (and elsewhere) to the problem of cultural appropriation might be seen as efforts to approach the world in better ways now that we – here, I especially mean white or white-passing liberals in the Euro-American orbit – can no longer credibly claim not to know anything about how we have approached the world *so far*.

As Sunila S. Kale and Christian Lee Novetzke define it,

The term "cultural appropriation" names the annexation by a dominant culture of some key elements of a minority culture in a context of unequal power ... Those making similar arguments about yoga posit that yoga has been appropriated by Western capitalism, dominated by a culture – almost homogenously white, upper middle class, capitalist, and consumerist – that valorizes a cisgender heteronormativity and is exemplified by an impossibly restrictive body type. In short: yoga has become controlled and corrupted by the most toxic of American cultural norms and, in the process, has lost its connections with the place of its origin, India … A key feature of the argument that presents [postural] yoga as a form of cultural appropriation asserts an explicit link between the contemporary Western colonization of yoga and the colonization of India by European powers.[48]

Critics often argue that modern postural yoga in the West too often approaches India and its religious and cultural products as though they can be consumed, reimagined, and merchandised by anyone for any reason. In *Yoga Makaranda* (1934), written long before cultural appropriation was on the societal radar in the West, the purported father of modern postural yoga, Krishnamacharya, anticipated the dynamics that Kale and Novetzke trace:

The foreigners have stolen all the skills and knowledge and treasures of mother India, either right in front of us or in a hidden way. They pretend that they have discovered all this by themselves, bundle it together, and then bring it back here as though doing us a favour and in exchange take all the money and things we have saved up for our family's welfare. After some time passes, they will try and do the same thing with *yogavidya* [the science/knowledge of yoga].

We can clearly state that the blame for this is that while we have read the books required for the knowledge of yoga to shine, we have not understood or studied the concepts or brought them into our experience. If we still sleep and keep our eyes closed, then the foreigners will become our gurus in *yogavidya*. We have already given the gold vessels we had to them and bought vessels from them made from bad-smelling skin and have started using these. This is a very sad state. Our descendants do not need these sorts of bad habits.[49]

Predictably, a broad sensitivity to the historical legacy of colonialism has created opportunities not just for dialogue but also for opportunism. Many yoga teachers, social media influencers, the Indian government, and groups such as the Hindu American Foundation have leapt into this space. Naturally, the political motives, financial interests, and social consequences of such gestures are often opaque to those in the target audience(s). For example, the Take Yoga Back campaign, organized by the Hindu American Foundation, is intended both to ensure that North American postural yoga is not divorced from its Indic origins and to boost India's stature in the international cultural arena.[50] Indian Prime Minister Narendra Modi's creation of the International Day of Yoga in 2014 reminds people of the Indic roots of yoga. But it also drafts the United Nations as well as individual nations into an apparently nonpolitical gesture that – probably not coincidentally – promotes the nationalist agenda of Modi's Bharatiya Janata Party. Similarly, podcasts such as *Yoga Is Dead* reflect informal campaigns by Indian American activists to protest insensitive or offensive uses of Indian religious or cultural practices or objects by yoga teachers, students, and studios.[51]

Certainly, many of the teachers I have met make sincere efforts to learn Sanskrit (or at least to pay close attention to the key texts and terms in the yogic tradition), to pronounce words correctly, to dress respectfully when they travel and teach, to take or send students to India to work with senior teachers, and to actively seek out teachers trained in India. Nonetheless, even if these efforts to underline the Indic origins of yoga are fairly well intentioned, they are also sometimes clumsy.[52]

One of the constant refrains in teacher-training programs and elsewhere in yogaland is the claim that there is a thick, unbroken, 5,000-year historical line connecting modern postural yoga in the West with ancient South Asian religion or philosophy. As we can see from the debates that surrounded Mark Singleton's *Yoga Body* (2010), it was once controversial to claim that the roots of postural yoga include cultural forms (e.g., body building and European exercise regimes) that have very little to do with Patanjali, Svatmarama, and Vivekananda.[53] But as scholar-practitioner Theodora Wildcroft observes in her book on "post-lineage yoga," "Among long-term yoga practitioners, there is a growing awareness that practices considered to be 'traditional' are in many cases modern inventions, or at least, radical reinterpretations of older practices."[54]

This newer account has not crowded out the 5,000-year-old origin story in yogaland, but over the years, students and teachers have shown less and less resistance to the distinctively modern Krishnamacharya-era origins of many of the postures and certainly of the set sequences. Claims about the long history of asana practices – connecting Indus Valley artifacts from thousands of years before the Common Era with activities in a contemporary Arkansas YMCA – might be inaccurate, but they tell us something important. The hope that the yoga practised in Arkansas actually emerged in sacred time immemorial (with Shiva often identified as the first yogi) represents both an indictment of the available religious, spiritual, and well-being options in the West and an expression of the sweetness, power, and solace that practitioners see in these Indic ideas and practices.

Now that I have sketched some of the backdrop of these debates, we can reflect on what the people I interviewed said when our discussions turned to cultural appropriation.

As a senior teacher in the Dharma Mittra yoga community argued, "I respect the history, but I feel [that] to make it relatable to people, so people can digest it, I need to make it universal." Joanne, an established Iyengar teacher in Vancouver, similarly noted, "I mean, Mr Iyengar was very clear on yoga being for all religions, and [he also argued] that it's a spiritual practice, not so much a religious practice. And so that supports me in my picking and choosing, you know, how I can interpret some of these [asanas and instructions]." Monica, an Iyengar teacher in Winnipeg, underlined this insight when she contended, "Cultural appropriation is not an issue in Iyengar yoga because yoga is … universal culture. It doesn't matter if you're white, if you're whatever, doesn't matter, your race, your creed, anything: it's universal culture. It's for you to figure out who you are, and that's right from the *Yoga Sutras* of Patanjali. It's a universal culture. I can't remember which sutra it's from."

One Dharma Mittra yoga student in Canada, Cathy, acknowledged that her approach to cultural appropriation reflects her own social location:

The first thing that I think of, and this might just be a total cop out, is that as a Canadian, I feel like most things are cultural appropriation. I don't know Ukrainian traditions very well, or Polish or Irish or Scottish or English or French [she is a mix of all]. I mean, everything's so globalized now. I don't know that I'm the best person to answer that because I am the middle-aged white woman, I mean, I'm *Cathy*. I'm no expert, I'm not a guru – I'm simply someone who wants to share the positive things that I've learned.[55]

Isabel, a vinyasa teacher in Indianapolis, said that she did not feel burdened by the dilemma of cultural appropriation: "I think at the end of the day, we're all people. We all want something. And [yoga is about] just like sensing that and showing up for each other. For me … I get [that Indian] culture is a part of [yoga], but it's just really about kindness and giving people hope and just all remembering we're all special. At the end of the day, we're all just trying to move our bodies and feel better."

Karen, a former Ashtanga teacher, noted, "I really want to kind of distill the whole practice … You know, I can peel away all the Sanskrit, I can peel away all of that. Because isn't it kind of universal when you study religion, that ultimately, isn't it about that kind of coming to a place of not harming?" Julie, a teacher in New York, agreed, arguing that we should relax our concerns about who owns what since in the grand scheme of things, "we're literally all the same thing. We're all one thing."

Rinku, a Torontonian teacher of South Asian descent, said, "When I first started to go to studios [eight years ago] and hear white teachers, [I would feel] there's just something about my culture that was taken away, and then it's like so expensive for me to access now. And then it's just like the pronunciation is just like not on point. But now at this point, I don't really look at it." Although her approach was less strident than it once had been, she noted how much the older Indian women she knew appreciated when a white teacher wore a sari: "When they see like a white person practising their culture, they're very proud. They're like, 'Oh look at you! You know, my daughter doesn't even wear a sari.'"

A few people I met were somewhat more defensive when the issue arose. Bart, a leader in the Canadian Ashtanga community, contended, "I give myself a pass on all this stuff. [Whenever people raise the issue of cultural appropriation, I say,] 'Like, hey man, I went there, I studied ten years. This is what my teachers told me to do.'" Ruth, a teacher in Toronto, echoed Bart when she made reference to what I have called an authorizing discourse:

I really take a lot of pride in where I received my training [Rishikesh]. I also have a lot of reverence for yoga, for the history, for the philosophy, for its cultural relevance, but also its religious relevance in India. And also, you know, because I learned [vinyasa] yoga in the birthplace of yoga. Like Rishikesh is the place where they discovered the first yoga text, so I have no reservations about saying the word namaste. I come back from India, and suddenly there are yoga studio owners telling me I'm not allowed to say namaste at the end of my class. Hmm. I'm like, "What are you talking about? I learned yoga in India and, and this is what I was taught. Why would I do anything other than what I was taught?" So my, my mentality has always been I want to pay homage to yoga in as pure of a way as I can. Not because I believe that I am Indian or Hindu in any way. But because I don't want to desecrate this thing that I didn't create.

John, a hatha teacher in Vancouver, said, "I don't think chanting [in Sanskrit] is cultural appropriation. I'm doing it within the culture of the traditions of yoga. It's not owned by Indian people. In fact, they brought it west so it would become popular. They were charged with going out west and spreading yoga to people [and they were successful in doing that]." Indeed, Marianne, a hot yoga teacher in Winnipeg, drew attention to the other motives behind debates around cultural appropriation: "I feel like maybe when cultural appropriation comes up, it's [paired with] this idea of purity and what's pure, what's real, like authentic. And you know, a lot of people love Ashtanga or love Iyengar [for this reason] – because they think it's pure, authentic. [They will say,] 'An Indian dude, you know, gave it to us; therefore,' et cetera, et cetera [sighs]. For me … there's no such thing as purity."

Public discourse around cultural appropriation is now well advanced, and there are well-established speedy reactions that one can anticipate when someone shows up to a Halloween party pretending to be a gay, disabled, Indigenous, or African American person. Still, Marianne's comment captures the sense in which North American yoga is becoming "more and more its own thing," as a teacher from Los Angeles said. In such a scenario, cultural appropriation is not really a problem since one cannot appropriate what is already one's own. No one we spoke with denied that appropriation was worth discussing, but as Kale and Novetzke point out, the situation is complicated. "If the measure of cultural appropriation is the very fact that yoga as a global phenomenon appears to be a Western one at this stage in history, then yoga has been appropriated by the West, although often with the explicit efforts of Indians, such as Pattabhi Jois, B.K.S. Iyengar, Bikram Choudhury, and a thriving yoga tourism industry in India."[56]

Cultural appropriation was certainly a topic about which all of the people I met had thought and one that they were able to discuss in some depth. However, the overall tone of these discussions was far more muted than I had anticipated. I had expected people to have strong opinions, but no matter how I approached the issue, almost no one seemed especially animated. This impression was also echoed in the survey results. When I asked about how people felt when teachers and students "used South Asian terms, imagery, and concepts without providing historical or philosophical context," 44 per cent said that they were not bothered at all, and another 36 per cent said that they were slightly bothered but not enough to bring it up with others.[57]

For some, the question of cultural appropriation was not vexing because, as Marianne commented, "I don't care to try to reverse the passing of time and try to make [the yoga that I teach and practise here] become more authentic to India. Heavy air quotes. Because it's not [Indian]. It's a North American form." Even practitioners for whom the Indian elements of the practice were still important for their own experience – or, if they were teachers, for their teaching – felt that they had already sincerely adopted an appropriately respectful approach to these features of yoga.

Conclusion

Throughout yogaland, we see a carefully selected Indian aesthetic in the use of incense, music, artwork, and statues; an Indian rhetoric in the adoption of asana names and Sanskrit chants; and an Indian worldview in references to samsara (the cycle of birth, death, and rebirth), samskaras (patterns of thought about ourselves based on our memories), karma (cause and effect), moksha (liberation), and samadhi (meditative absorption); an Indian deference to one's teacher; and an Indian calendar in which events such as Navaratri, Holi, Diwali, and moon days are sometimes observed.

It is not difficult to see not only how India is constructed in the minds of students and teachers as a magical, timeless, beautiful antidote to vapid Western societies that are too loud, fast, and dirty but also how it is then used to support what we might consider the understandable authenticity projects of studios, lineages, teachers, students, clothing lines, workshops, and styles. As a symbol or state of mind more than a nation-state, India is a load-bearing wall of modern postural yoga in North America.

Two crises seem to have challenged this stature.

First, for people who identified with figures such as Pattabhi Jois, Muktananda, Vishnudevananda, Amrit Desai, Yogi Bhajan, Satchidananda, Manouso Manos, and Bikram Choudhury – to name just a few – the #MeToo scandals raised harrowing questions. How did it come to pass that so many people tolerated their problematic behaviour – ranging from appalling to inappropriate – for so long? How have so many of the men remained, even after some of their deaths, in positions of real or symbolic power in their communities? What explains the often equivocal and ambivalent responses of former students *today*? Why are there still garlands around photos of deceased and disgraced teachers *today*? Why the "guru*ji*" *today*?

The past few years within yogaland have revealed how many unscrupulous teachers took advantage of often vulnerable or traumatized students. Desperate for remedies that they could not access anywhere else, practitioners found themselves in terrible situations – and some may still feel trapped. Although there is no way to undo the pain already inflicted by predators and their enablers, practitioners now have both an opportunity and a responsibility to ask questions about the social forces within their communities that may have built or reinforced the protective walls around these figures.

Here, we can intuit the link to a second crisis.

With unprecedented access to information about the often dark history of North America (as we see with the report of Canada's Truth and Reconciliation Commission), it has become more difficult to assume any kind of superiority over other societies. But naive fantasies about other communities are more difficult to sustain too. Yes, yogaland has been encumbered by Orientalism since and of course before Vivekananda took the podium at Chicago's World Parliament of Religions in 1893.[58] And yes, India continues to be portrayed as essentially exotic in popular culture, as we see in Elizabeth

Gilbert's book *Eat, Pray, Love* (2006), in its film adaptation of 2010,[59] and indeed in many Bollywood films.

But change is afoot. Due to fairly affordable international travel and to the increasingly diverse ethnocultural profile of North America's cities, where people of South Asian descent have put down deep roots, India has lost some of its mystique; in this sense, it is an increasingly ordinary country. It is now hard not to cringe at the naive Orientalist projections of the excited North Americans who first welcomed figures such as Vivekananda, Muktananda, Paramahansa Yogananda, and Osho or, more recently, Bikram and Jois. Cultural appropriation was simply easier when one knew very little about either one's own privileges or the cultural practice or object being appropriated. It was easier when one's neighbours were unlikely to frown upon one's unprincipled or even naive borrowing.

Earlier in this chapter, I mentioned that it was not at all obvious that yoga in Canada and the United States would survive sex scandals *and* a growing awareness of the problematic ways that yogaland profits from South Asian religious and cultural appropriation. For practitioners living in a time and subculture in which cultural safety, equity, diversity, and multiculturalism are much-lauded values, it is deeply distressing to learn not just that yoga communities are not citadels of sexual integrity but also that by listening to a podcast by a white teacher about career strategies derived from the *Bhagavad Gita*, one might be an unwitting participant in the trivialization of a great, yet beleaguered, civilization.

But even with the ignominy of #MeToo and the deep awkwardness created by debates over cultural appropriation, yoga persists. Certainly, the people I met gave me the impression that the recent reconfiguration of the studios in North American cities is not the result of the two crises that I have teased out here but the result of the economic impact of a three-year pandemic. The two crises discussed in this chapter have in fact had major, although rather ambiguous, impacts on yogaland. Given North American yoga's wide range of styles, practice contexts, costs, and audiences – some with no ties to any lineage and some with direct ties to major twentieth- and twenty-first-century gurus – it should be no surprise that we see a diversity of responses to sexual misconduct and cultural appropriation. This mixed response means that India, as a notion and a nation, also continues to be invoked in a wide variety of ways.

This range allows people to pick and choose. If one does not feel the need to understand the language in which one chants mantras, there are options. If one wants to go to India to practice yoga, learn Sanskrit, and volunteer in orphanages, there are options. If one does not like to be surrounded by photos of a Speedo-clad "boss," there are options. If one seeks studios where all teachers are beautiful white women who end each class with the greeting namaste, there are options. If one feels that although gurus have been shown to be flawed, they are healers who still deserve to be venerated, there are options. If one rejects cultural appropriation and misogyny but feels that these concerns have been resolved, there are options. And if one feels that we are in the midst of the Kali Yuga (age of decline) and that the scandals are birth pangs of a new world, there are options too.

Shavasana

One day in Los Angeles, an Ashtanga teacher asked sixteen of us to come to the top of our mats in a large airy room on the second floor of a commercial building. This is always one of my favourite moments in a led practice. I know that I am about to join others in doing something difficult and wonderful, and finally, after more than a decade of committed practice, I have a decent sense of what to do. I looked past the teacher and out the window behind her, where I could see the Pacific Ocean through the palm trees. I drew my attention from the natural splendour of California into the room, where I allowed my drishti (gaze) to wander. I took in the well-coordinated clothing, the expensive mats, and the cork floor. I admired the taut, tanned, and tattooed bodies and equanimous faces of people I would never meet again, but who were, for the next ninety minutes, kin. We would breathe and move together, and then we would return to our lives.

The teacher waited for all of us to settle into samasthiti (equal standing pose). There we waited, hands at heart centre, eyes closed, expecting her to begin the opening chant. Once the room was silent, she did something teachers almost never do. She asked, "What is the most difficult asana?" We all looked at her over the tips of our fingers.

One student at the front of the class answered, "Kapotasana?" – the pigeon pose (see figure C.1) – assuming that the deep backbend, with knees bent, shins and forearms on the ground, and one's hands on the bottoms of one's feet, would be a likely candidate. "Oh god, yes! Kapo's brutal," a possible supermodel to my left whispered. I had only been given the first few postures from the Ashtanga intermediate series and privately hoped that my teachers would know better than to ask me to try this one.

The teacher smiled, tilted her head slightly, and asked, "Anyone else?"

A practitioner in the middle of the room said, "Vrishchikasana, no question" – referring to the scorpion pose (see figure C.2). An inversion with one's weight balanced on parallel forearms, combined with a backbend in which one's feet touch one's head, it is a wonder to behold. A student in Indianapolis referred to it as "very Cirque du Soleil."

"Anyone else?"

We had figured out the trick. "Shavasana?" (corpse pose) a fidgety student at the back of the room offered.

"Yes, exactly. It can be hard, though not impossible, to have profound insights when we are trying to do complicated things with our bodies. That's why shavasana is so hard – because we don't get to be distracted from what Patanjali meant by citta vritti – all the fluctuations of the mind."

She let that sink in. "Okay. Now, let's breathe." After four breaths, we intoned, "Om," chanted the opening invocation, "Vande Gurunam ...," and we were off.

As I inhaled and raised my hands high above my head for the first surya namaskara (sun salutation pose), I thought about how these Californians would have puzzled ancient Patanjali, late medieval Svatmarama, and likely even modern Tirumalai Krishnamacharya. My focus in this book has not been the history of yoga but the meanings that contemporary North Americans give to this practice. As I mentioned earlier, I am interested in determining not what yoga really is but what it also is.

There are moments in a studio – when non-Sanskrit readers chant Sanskrit mantras, when students treat their teachers with extreme reverence, or when teachers stand right beside a statue of Ganesh and say that the practice has nothing to do with religion – when the distinctive features of contemporary yoga really stand out. Now that we are entering the shavasana phase,

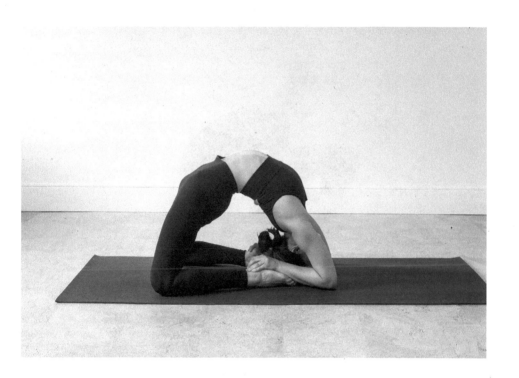

Figure C.1
Kapotasana (pigeon pose)

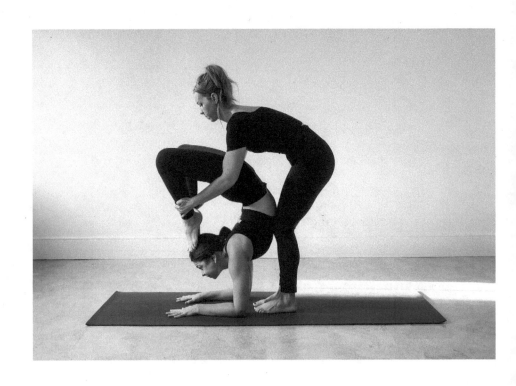

Figure C.2
Vrishchikasana (scorpion pose)

we can pause to integrate what we have learned about these people, their practices, and the societies that shape postural yoga today.

First, however, I should note that I was, and am, one of these people.

For the past two decades, I have obeyed the expected professional manners of yogaland and kept my personal experiences more or less to myself. I certainly referred to myself (as a non-Christian) when writing about evangelical Christians in 2000, and I have also referred to myself (as the son of a racialized immigrant) when writing about migration policy and multiculturalism since about 2005. Including these kinds of reflections has become increasingly acceptable as a means of expressing one's "positionality" (to use one of the uglier words that academics have coined in the past few decades). Nonetheless, in the early decades of my career, I would mention the particularities of my life as little as possible. I do not think that I really treated my interiority, my affective states, my all-too-human ego striving, or my physical ailments as integral parts of what I was learning, writing, and teaching.

By the end of my fieldwork period, I came to feel that it makes no sense to set aside insights that I have collected with my mind and body during more than a decade of yoga practice and study.

The reality – from my vantage point at least – is that although there is, in some ways, more openness to multiple perspectives in universities now than ever before, a strong suspicion about subjective data remains. To use one's life experience as data is to open one up to ridicule from those who maintain that personal material pollutes everything and should either be used as an amusing anecdote in a book's foreword or preferably avoided altogether. The problem that my peers intuit in the increasing openness to subjective data is captured well in a maxim attributed to Anaïs Nin. Her observation is over sixty years old, but it has circulated far and wide through social media in the past decade. "We do not see things as they are, we see them as we are," she wrote.[1] I appreciate the cautionary tone of her insight, but I also think that we can engage our shared world in a manner that is not entirely bound by our origins and idiosyncrasies.

When I noted in the book's introduction that I am an insider and an outsider in this project, I assumed that readers would think that the inside in question refers to my yoga life. That is true, but of course, I am also inside the academy, an environment that is as rule-bound as any yoga space. (If you doubt that, just audit any honours seminar at any research-intensive university.) Although I have tried to be self-critical about my yoga insiderness, I also want to be self-critical about my academic insiderness.

Both yogaland and universityland are spaces with long histories and complicated relationships to the societies that produced them and to the people who fill their classes. The rules that govern yoga and scholarly spaces emerged over centuries to protect the power structures and communal norms of these spaces. That is exactly as one would expect, but it is helpful to remember that the cultural trends, financial pressures, and power politics that shape the contemporary university are partially hidden from ordinary members of these communities, just as neither the inner workings nor the external pressures of yogaland are visible to all practitioners. Yogaland and universityland also share the sense that the world as it appears to us may not be actually how it is. Both places can be critical and life-giving, just as both can be bulwarks in the lonely, planet-killing, soul-destroying status quo.

As well, I should repeat something that I emphasized in the first few pages: this book is not about me, or at least I hope not. I leaned on existing research, and I conducted new research, but more than that, my interactions with practitioners and scholars from around the world suggest that the basic argument might travel too.

Beyond What You Told Them

Readers might have heard the advice that professors, pastors, and politicians often receive from mentors about a formula for good speaking or writing: tell people what you are going to tell them, tell them, and then tell them what you told them. I do not think that it would be very interesting to recapitulate all of the findings when they are more thoroughly explored in the previous pages. Nonetheless, I think that it might be worthwhile to reflect on a few issues that straddle the whole book.[2]

CONCLUSION

Cosmopolitans Come Home

I began this project almost exclusively interested in the ways that postural yoga might be influenced by the societies – specifically the nations – in which it flourishes. I did ultimately broaden my focus. Nonetheless, I can confirm what many practitioners will know, namely that most North American (indeed, also western European) yoga spaces do indeed look and feel quite similar. Virtually all of them share a common aesthetic and create a common anti-world atmosphere. However, practitioners generally did not talk about explicitly political concerns without being nudged.

As appealing as it is to imagine that North Americans and western Europeans inhabit a common borderless, cosmopolitan, liberal arena, individuals actually live in specific neighbourhoods, cities, and societies.[3] Nobody lives nowhere, in other words. The United States and Canada share many things, but they are certainly distinguishable when it comes to gun culture, race-related discourses, political polarization, and the often precarious situations of women and LGBTQIA+ citizens. Canada is by no means a paradise, but on these issues, there are meaningful differences.[4]

But as is clear as soon as friends and colleagues from the United States and Canada compare notes, probably the most dramatic discrepancy between these two societies is their approach to health care. In chapter 3, I noted that Canadians do often complain about the accessibility and efficiency of its "single-payer" health system, but it would be political suicide for a major political party to advocate replacing it with an American-style system. By the end of our fieldwork, the project research assistant (an American anthropologist) had become accustomed to seeing my Canada face, which would appear whenever American participants told stories (and most of them had such accounts to share) about a life-altering medical bill or an argument with an insurance agent responsible for decisions that would lead to very different health outcomes.

Wellness interventions such as yoga mean slightly different things depending on the ways that a given society imagines (and funds) health care, of course. But although the health care system on which one is dependent matters a great deal, the broader lesson is that we need to factor what I have called meso- or national-level realities into our understandings of why people might seek healing through alternative or complementary modalities such as yoga, reiki, acupuncture, Ayurvedic medicine, massage, and meditation.

Concepts and Conflicts

Claims articulated about religion or spirituality often seem invulnerable to critique. That is especially true when the claims appear in the legal or media arenas or if they appear to relate to very private matters such as sexuality or death. The reticence that many of us feel about asking follow-up questions about such claims often cuts short very productive conversations. This tendency is unfortunate since in many cases it prevents us from understanding why certain people come to hold certain views in certain places and times.

In our survey, for example, 92.8 per cent of respondents said that their yoga practice was spiritual.[5] That is a very high percentage, and quite interesting, but such comments ought to be the beginning of a conversation, not the end. The categories of religious and spiritual – and their cousins secular, sacred, agnostic, atheist, liberal, and so on – are not merely convenient labels. They are not like the words cupboard, antelope, or cabbage, the meanings of which are not often the subject of serious dispute. In contrast, in my field, debates over the meanings of religion, spirituality, and their cousins inspire books, special issues of journals, and – believe it or not – departmental schisms.

When people declare, "Yoga is …," they are not just talking about yoga. In fact, sometimes they are hardly talking about yoga at all.[6] Such claims often reveal a great deal about what they think about Asia, their bodies, their families, their traumas, and their society's health care system. Anyone interested in understanding yoga practitioners, the subcultures that they have created, and the cultures that have created them, should pay close attention to claims about the more-than-physical aspects of the practice. We need to take them seriously, although not literally.

The same thing goes for India, which in yogaland is not just a state with a certain population, climate, and political system. Thanks to the scale and richness of the civilization that Europeans encountered hundreds of years ago when they set their sights on the subcontinent, it was possible for mystics, merchants, bohemians, and benefactors to find whatever they were looking for in what we might think of as the Rorschach test that is South Asia. The aura surrounding India and its vast spiritual resources is essential for the success of postural yoga. Without it, "all we're doing is exercise," as one student noted.

There is a lot at stake for insiders when they think, talk, and dream about India, samadhi (meditative absorption), or authenticity. These powerful metaphors are used to situate modern postural yoga within a tradition typically framed as timeless, anti-materialistic, and spiritual.

Many of the people I met in order to write this book attribute religious or spiritual meanings to postural yoga, but obviously there are practitioners who are religiously "unmusical," a phrase that Max Weber used as a self-description.[7] For them, yoga is a fitness activity that takes place in a space with an Indic aesthetic. They give these features no more thought than they do the antique shovels and sombreros that hang on the walls of the Tex-Mex pub that they might visit on Friday after work.

I do not want this observation and analogy to sound dismissive. One of the key teachings of many forms of yoga – or for that matter, many spiritual and religious traditions – is captured in the adage "Every head contains a world."[8] Even complete indifference to practices and philosophies with deep roots in past and present capital-R religions tells us something about the human capacity to compartmentalize and to see one's own world as the only world. It is true, of course, that we each have the power to imagine and sustain comprehensive and idiosyncratic accounts of the world. But these heads do not independently produce these worlds. They sit atop bodies that live and breathe in particular societies, geographies, legal systems, economies, families, and religious institutions. These political, material, and cultural facts shape the worlds that are created and shared with others. These forces prevail upon me too, situated as my head and body are in a particular country, social class, ethnoracial and linguistic context, and time in history.

The tendencies captured in the previous paragraph are perfectly suited to the culture of therapeutic individualism,[9] which frames everything in terms most convenient to the modern consumer. Whether the capacity to bracket the Indic aspects of postural yoga in pursuit of personal wellness reflects a post-modern form of spirituality is not for me to determine (at least not here), but it certainly is indicative of North American society.

Fragile Bodies in a Hostile World

Those who remain involved in yoga practice after their initial physical complaints are addressed tend to be interested in studios either as sites of social interaction or as contexts in which they can learn to diminish the damage inflicted by a loud, fast, and dirty world. Patanjali would agree with Bessel van der Kolk that "the body keeps the score,"[10] partly because the mind, like the larger culture that informs the body, encourages it to do exactly that.

But in studios another promise is made, one that is often just whispered and often only subconsciously grasped by teachers, namely that the bruised, belaboured, and besmirched body might also *settle* the score. Within this promise is a critique, maybe an indictment, of the conventional tools that our societies offer us to repair the damage that the world does to us.

Throughout this book, we have seen how practitioners often frame yoga as a means to help fragile bodies to cope with a hostile world. I have argued that the national (or meso) forces are as important as the personal and local (or micro) forces in explaining the anti-world of postural yoga. That should not distract us from the fact that our bodies are embedded in a world beset by global (or macro) forces so large and menacing that our imaginations can hardly comprehend either the true nature of the threat or the appropriate remedies.

In the summer of 2023, as I was writing this book, the world was in the middle of the hottest year in recorded history, with droughts, forest fires, and floods filling our news feeds and nightmares. As I now near the end of my writing in 2024, a new war rages between Israel and Palestine, the result of which will almost certainly be further devastation and despair in the region. The war between Russia and Ukraine is no longer in the international news every day, but it continues to cause tremendous suffering and dislocation. Conflicts and crises are rampant.

These global forces seem very far removed from what might happen in a studio or at home on a mat. But it is a feature of modernity, or perhaps postmodernity, that more than ever before, our lives combine here and there, now and then, and later. So not all traumas are local or immediate. Some come at us through nonstop exposure to an unravelling world: the dark predictions of the United Nations Intergovernmental Panel on Climate Change, haunting images of boats overflowing with refugees in the Mediterranean Sea, grotesque videos of hospitals, kibbutzim, and daycares with bloody floors, and aerial footage of neighbourhoods transformed into rubble. All of these facts leave their marks on our bodies too. My sense is that practitioners concerned about the climate crisis or humanitarian disasters experience yoga either as an escape from an impending cataclysm or as a way to make them strong and flexible enough to survive the traumas that it seems the future will bring.[11] Or perhaps yoga is both at the same time.

Enchantment and Its Discontents

I reflect on enchantment in two ways. First, it is rather peculiar that the mind reading, time travelling, and shape-shifting that we find in Patanjali's *Yoga Sutras* are almost never mentioned in contemporary yoga settings, on the one hand, and that the asanas that many North Americans consider to be the sine qua non of postural yoga are almost entirely absent from the same text, on the other hand.

Although scholars and practitioners agree by tacit consensus not to talk (almost at all) about superpowers or (very much) about the conspicuous absence of asanas in the *Yoga Sutras*, spiritual beings are still present in shalas today. Of course, figures such as the lithe Krishnamacharya, the timeless Babaji, the ineffable Ramana, and the divine Shiva exist on the walls and in the lore of yogaland, but I am referring to the preternaturally gifted, charismatic contemporary students and teachers who often become the focal points of postural yoga communities.

The physical beauty and athletic grace of these siddhas (perfected beings) – a term that I use very loosely – is a necessary but not sufficient cause of their prestige. One could say that, being gifted at asana practice but also able to articulate yogic philosophy, these individuals speak volumes with their enchanted and enchanting bodies. In the most literal sense, these jivanmuktas (superpeople) embody promises made by yoga traditions for centuries: one can be liberated from one's body through one's body while still in one's body.[12] Their powers are rarely discussed, but these beguiling and exceptional superhumans are often at the still centre of many communities. You will know them when you see them because it will be difficult to look away.

Enchantment arose in a second way too. One throughline in research on religion is the threat that critical research is assumed to pose to the convictions, communities, and practices of deep insiders. Disenchantment is a danger with a great deal of research, of course. Consider the professor of English who no longer reads for pleasure because their professional interest in the ideological features of novels has waged a successful war with the unadulterated joy that they once felt as a child, curled up on a couch, innocently engrossed in J.R.R. Tolkien's *The Lord of the Rings*.

When I decided to apply my academic training to yoga, I worried about such an outcome. I thought that there was a real possibility that my commitment to the scholarly approach to religion, spirituality, and yoga would mean that one day my alarm would go off at 5:00 a.m., and I would not just hit the snooze button but give up on my early mornings at the shala altogether. I mentioned in the book's introduction that I did not want to become that guy who moves to the West Coast, takes up yoga, becomes a vegan, and buys a kayak. I am now mostly that guy (minus the vegan part). But I also did not want to become that other guy: the one whose disciplined approach to thinking about religion ruins any chance of having religious experiences. If my academic peers find the category of religious experience to be overloaded or inert, they can substitute cognate terms such as spiritual, ecstatic, ineffable, or mystical instead. The point is that I did not want to make such experiences – whatever word one might use to describe them – impossible.

There was nonetheless good reason to be suspicious about whether a personal commitment to yoga might distract me from the ways that both my own practice and the practices of others are shaped by social, economic, psychological, ethnoracial, or ideological interests and biases. In my view, the normal facts of my life – including my gender, nationality, social class, and age – influence my experience of and approach to yoga, but this influence does not make me unusual since nothing escapes these shaping forces. I am just not convinced that the spiritual, religious, or mystical experiences that I have heard about, witnessed, and had myself are entirely reducible to these facts.

I began practising yoga late in 2013 with no interest in it as a scholarly topic. It was the controversy that raged over the proposed 2015 closure of a Vancouver bridge for the first International Day of Yoga that made me want to think and write systematically about this peculiar phenomenon. I can now report – with some surprise, to be honest – that even with a more recent period of intensive fieldwork, my practice has become not just more interesting but more meaningful to me. I am still a skeptic, but that is a personality trait rather than a personal accomplishment. I remain grateful that the skepticism has not yet flattened the experiences that I am able to have or dulled my appreciation of what I think of as the "Amazing Grace" stories that are so common in yogaland – and indeed in many other religious, spiritual, and political communities.

Now that I have talked at length with practitioners, completed a teacher-training course, assessed our survey, and engaged in over a decade of study and practice, I no longer experience or think about yoga as I once did. Partly, that is because the many personal traumas that practitioners shared with me deepened my appreciation of just how well yoga seems to address a world that is painfully loud, fast, and dirty for so many people. And partly, it is because my approach to yoga has been changed by learning far more than I had anticipated about the doggedly romantic views that practitioners have of Asia, about the mixed messages sent to students concerning their bodies, about the rivalries between asana lineages and styles, about the way that the yoga economy chews up so many teachers, and about the troubling presence of "conspirituality" in yogaland.[13] Each of these influences has shifted my thinking in different directions, of course, but the cumulative effect has been that my practice and understanding of yoga are no longer as innocent as they were in 2013. This outcome is entirely predictable and even desirable.

As carefully curated as yoga spaces are, these anti-worlds are never free from the regular world's tribulations. To put it another way: survival in a period of political and climate crises is a project, a predicament. The odds are against most of us. After all, the dominant society militates against practices of introspection and also against a more radical political critique that might change the local, national, and global conditions that generate most suffering in the first place. It is hardly surprising that imperilled soft animals like those invoked in Mary Oliver's famous poem,[14] increasingly threatened by forces that are personal, political, and environmental, are drawn to spaces carefully crafted to be what one might fairly describe as "the heart of a heartless world and the soul of soulless conditions."[15]

But annihilation of or escape from such conditions might not be the only options. Perhaps a sober assessment of the social forces that are present in and behind yogaland makes a case for what I have called a yoga for adults. This notion might also underline my understanding of adulthood: a state of mind in which one can subject one's commitments and communities to critical scrutiny and yet remain involved with such ideas, practices, and people even after the end of innocence.

Metaphors and Me

Practitioners often say that yoga works on both sthula (gross) and sukshma (subtle) bodies. Working methodically toward the right relationship between the two is a central component in one's movement in the direction of kaivalya. In the yogi's subtle body, prana (the inward and upward energy mentioned in the *Yoga Sutras*) might meet apana (the downward and outward energy). In shavasana, one might grasp both viscerally and intuitively the relationship between one's atman (higher self) and Brahman (ultimate reality). Perhaps kundalini (the serpentine energy coiled at the base of the spine) might be aroused and in so doing enable some kind of transcendence. The promotion of a comprehensive and consistent Indic model of the mind and body is not the explicit agenda of most asana communities. Yet it seems to me that the model is still there, sublimated but available, as is briefly evident in innocent comments heard in many studios about chakras, karma, prana, shakti, bindu, nadis, kriyas, and samadhi.

I do not use these metaphors very often or unironically in my own practice or teaching, although that is not because I reject the possibility that there might be something akin to a subtle body with its own anatomy and physiology. Rather, I cannot quite shake the sense that the eager uptake of these terms in the West is part of an acquisitive approach to South Asia, a region from which so much has been taken in the past several centuries. The situation is complicated, of course, because key figures such as Paramahansa Yogananda, Swami Vivekananda, and Tirumalai Krishnamacharya also actively offered yoga to the same societies that had expressed, to say the least, ambivalent feelings about Asia and Asians for so long.

As someone who is in a literal sense the product of global flows of Western and South Asian people animated by personal and imperial interests, I have reservations about adopting too wholeheartedly a spiritual or philosophical paradigm that is also part of the same flow. I have been moved by seeing others handle these metaphors with respect, and I benefit tremendously from them, whether they are invoked to help bolster physical health or are intended to aid mental health. I might find the metaphors more resonant later, but at this point I use them with caution and irony.

Although I feel at home in yogaland's anti-world, I cannot forget that the mat and the territory on which it sits are integrally related. These mats are located in rooms rented by businesspeople who need to cover their rent and market their services, in cities with safe and unsafe areas, in societies with opioid and suicide crises, in health systems run by medical specialists or corporations, in provinces or states where one language overshadows others, and in countries built by immigration, slavery, love, families, religion, capitalism, hope, and ambivalent feelings about colonialism. The mats are not (just) magic carpets: they are sites where powerful social and political forces meet deep spiritual and personal aspirations.

For example, most yogic traditions did not need to make an argument for the primacy of the male body and experience; it was simply presupposed for millennia. As old and powerful as these androcentric traditions are, it seems to me that in modern postural yoga spaces, the great men of yoga appear to have met their match. There were no banners or petitions, no legal challenges or sit-ins, no riots or public protests, but there was nonetheless a revolution between the time of Patanjali – even the time of Krishnamacharya – and the time of Kino MacGregor and Adriene Mishler.[16]

Male predators and pundits will continue to use yoga spaces for their own gratification, but just glance at the thousands of photographs from yoga retreats and teacher trainings on social media, and you will see the future. The new normal need not be exclusively governed by women, but there is no question that a fundamental shift has occurred, and men are not in charge of the transformation.

That might be very welcome news for many practitioners, but it sits awkwardly alongside the fact that yoga as a physical-spiritual-therapeutic practice fits quite well within a society that wants just one thing from all of us: *more*.

I hope others will continue to draw attention to the way the yogic anti-world often patches people up just so they can be sent right back into an economic system that casts humans as utility-maximizing competitors more and more alienated from one another and their own bodies. It is hard to know whether one day practitioners might become more comfortable talking about the political world in which we are all entangled, a world that produces the need for the balm of yoga in the first place. In some sense, it is not in the commercial interest of studio owners and teachers to encourage students to look beyond the innocent views of yoga sometimes promoted in yogaland, but if the world continues its slide toward the political and environmental Kali Yuga (age of decline) – as described in Hindu literature – these communities may yet take it upon themselves to connect shala and society in new ways.

Shala and Society

Amanda Lucia writes that "the yoga mat is a deeply personal intimate space carved out for personal spiritual introspection. For many practitioners, the yoga mat is not only a material object but also a physical space, a mental state, and a community of practitioners."[17] Given how many psychological, political, and economic forces are present on these roughly 12 square feet of vinyl, rubber, or cork, it is a wonder there is room for a human body as well. But it is in the body on the mat that these forces become apparent, and perhaps, if only briefly, the body is where they can be transcended through disciplined practice.

But what kind of body is this? Just as archaeologists scrape off the layers of old documents to find even older ones underneath, when we rub the surface of the gross body, we see other bodies – spiritual, imaginary, cultural, political, superhuman – and societies past and present, East and West, folded in on themselves. Within the accomplished, traumatized, or yearning adult, we also see the body and mind of the child. It may be the case that we are never free from the fears, enchantments, and certainties of children. But it may also be the core task of adulthood to struggle openly with ideas, feelings, and habits that might not be, and might never become, consistent. One of the main throughlines of this book has been the argument that thinking dispassionately about something you love passionately can both break your heart and free you to enter into that thing – yoga, America, Canada, your marriage, yourself – with open eyes and a posture of curiosity.

However, it is, of course, complicated. We use this word a lot, but its literal meaning is instructive: to fold together (from the Latin *com* and *plicare*), to combine in one concatenation of space and time far more than appears possible.[18] In these anti-worlds, we see folded, broken, luminous bodies seeking health, solace, solidarity, beauty, immortality, orthodoxy, and wholeness.

North American postural yoga practice invites students to do complicated things that once seemed unimaginable, from simply touching one's toes to crossing one's feet behind one's head to being quiet for an hour. Many students remember the first time they crossed a threshold with prasarita padottanasana C (wide-legged forward bend pose C; see figure C.3). In this standing posture, your legs are widely spread and your shoulders are rolled back. Your arms are straight, and your hands are clasped near your tailbone. Then you fold forward at the hips and try to rest your head on the floor between your legs while your hands – still clasped at the end of straight arms, mind you – are slowly brought to the floor a few feet behind your head, which, remember, is on the floor under your pelvis. It is a rather improbable posture to describe and see. Most students cannot touch the floor with their head and hands, even with the help of a good teacher, but when they do, it feels as though their hands might belong to someone else.

Several years ago, when Annie guided my hands to the floor for the first time, my mental picture of my body was completely at odds with the sensations my body was sending me. I broke form and stood up more quickly than usual, eyes wide open.

"Whoa. What just happened?" I asked.

Annie smiled beatifically, scrunching up her eyes as she whispered, "Good," and then stepped away.

When my mind integrated what my body had just done, I wondered how many other certitudes I did not need to grip so tightly.

I did not begin my practice with any intention to study it or to have it become the central feature of my professional or spiritual life. My interests were far more utilitarian, driven by desperation and pain. I suppose it was just good fortune that I found in these practices, and in these communities, both a new research direction and an effective approach to the liberation of my mind and body from burdens they do not need to carry anymore. That is why in the book's introduction I described the story I had to tell – notwithstanding my scholarly ambivalence – as a conversion story.

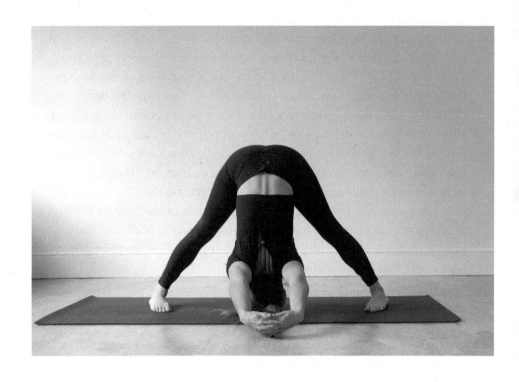

Figure C.3
Prasarita padottanasana C (wide-legged forward bend pose C)

At the Intersection
of Loud, Fast, and Dirty

Sometimes a posture feels impossible. Depending on how cooperative my joints are, sometimes the posture that seems most daunting is marichyasana D (ray of light pose D), and sometimes it is tittibhasana A (firefly pose A; see figure A.1), in which you balance the back of your thighs on your triceps, open your legs wide, point your toes, and suspend your weight entirely on your hands.

Every student has his or her tormenters. You try and try, but some days you just cannot get the bind or the balance, open your hips enough, regularize your breathing, or remember how to release the bind without falling over. Some teachers will say that you must keep trying before you learn other asanas. On other occasions, they will just observe the blockage and suggest that you return to the difficult posture later.

Academics often use the conclusion of a book to outline questions that merit future research. Since this book does not fit snugly within the conventional scholarly genre, I decided to reflect in a separate chapter on five questions that still need to be addressed. This is partly an appendix, partly a coda, and at the very end, partly a brief exploration of the higher purpose of asana practice.

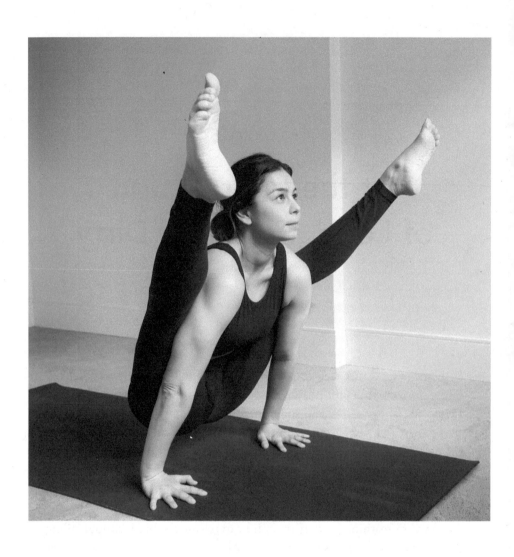

Figure A.1
Tittibhasana A (firefly pose A)

Transgender Inclusion

In Canada and in many US states, universities, school boards, hospitals, and other public employers have policies about pronoun use, washroom access, and other matters related to LGBTQIA+ community interests. Many professional sports leagues and entertainment corporations have also sought (clumsily, perhaps) to respond constructively. The issue has become a central feature of the so-called culture wars, especially in the United States, where the suppression of LGBTQIA+ rights is often used to signal loyalty to the most conservative parts of the Republican base.

The trans community is, of course, front and centre in these debates. Given the prominence of these concerns in so many places in North America, it was fascinating that trans-related issues almost never came up without me raising them in interviews or informal interactions. To be clear, when I did raise these topics, the responses were uniformly liberal, just as they were when I put race and cultural appropriation on the table, by which I mean that everyone agreed that trans people are entirely welcome.[1] These conversations did not last long because comments were nearly identical and broadly egalitarian regardless of how I raised the issue. To borrow a term from Scientology, the topic lacked "charge" whenever it was brought up, and so after a few efforts to elicit engagement, we moved on.

For me, however, the issue was still conspicuous by its absence or low profile in the public discourse of the communities that I visited. I was puzzled not just because this topic is a common and often controversial one in so many social spaces in North America but also because the body and its possible transformations are such central concerns in studios. Why are the staff of the Nova Scotia public service required to think more about trans inclusion than the staff and senior students of so many yoga spaces throughout North America?[2]

It was not until the final fifteen minutes of the final focus group of the seventh and final city visit that someone brought up trans inclusion without a prompt. In this case, the person mentioned their own positive experience as a trans practitioner. I asked for a separate interview with Sidney after the focus group. When I asked how they would explain why we had yet to hear people introduce these topics into our many (perhaps thousands) of hours of fieldwork, they offered a profound explanation:

I know a lot of trans people who box or who power lift or who [participate in activities] where it's not about turning inward and thinking and reflecting [which is, after all, one of] the [core] spiritual tenets of yoga. The idea of connecting with the self doesn't resonate [with trans people] for that very reason because the body is a source of distress. Um, so the [focus group] participant today who talked about hip openers and the kind of emotional release associated with that? [Well,] that is triggering for a lot of trans people [who are] not interested in having a public emotional release, um, in the hips or in any region that's connected to the pelvis. So, so yeah, there's something about the kind of movement and the invitation to check in with the body that yoga offers that I think is not a safe space for trans folks who are actively distressed in their embodiment.

Sidney highlights the difficulty they faced with the focus on pelvic anatomy given that (for them and their trans friends) the body is often a fraught space. Sidney has found a teacher whose touch they trust and who is careful about how she describes postures, but many people will not be so fortunate. Their story was a revelation to me, I confess. An even thornier issue that they face is the fact that yoga spaces lean on gender and sexual binaries, from male and female change rooms to references to Shiva and Shakti to yin and yang to purusha (consciousness) and prakriti (material nature). The list is long.

It seems to me that yogaland – with some exceptions, of course[3] – is near the beginning of a long and necessary conversation about what it means to include trans or gender-nonconforming people in yoga spaces. It will be interesting to observe and reflect on the ways that these issues are managed, especially since so many other sites in our societies began the conversation many years earlier.

Indigenous and African American Reconciliation

Indigenous issues are far more prominent concerns in Canadian public and political discourse than they are in the United States. This circumstance is predictable. In my country, the mistreatment of Indigenous people – especially children during the residential school period (1870s–1990s) – has been the topic of national inquiries, legal challenges, art exhibits, media exposés, government policies, university curriculum changes, and kitchen table debates for quite a while.[4]

The absence of Indigenous themes in the ordinary give and take of my conversations with practitioners was most conspicuous in Winnipeg, with a population that is 15 to 20 per cent Indigenous.[5] Similar processes are at work in the US yoga scene, where the very low number of nonwhite participants mostly goes, as it were, without saying. There, the Black Lives Matter movement was hardly mentioned, although the cities that we visited have sizable and marginalized African American populations.[6]

As in the case of cultural appropriation and trans issues, any comments that were shared in response to prompts on these themes were reliably positive and liberal. It is nonetheless still interesting that Canadian and American practitioners did not on their own connect their practices with the key racial justice movements in their respective societies. The limited prominence within yogaland of racial justice considerations is a reminder of the ways that inherited privileges make it difficult even for conscientious people to see, much less critique, the advantages they have. What might need to happen within yogaland or in the surrounding societies to alter this approach to minority communities?

Yogaland after COVID-19

It is not as though teachers first became aware of the often grim financial dimensions of the yoga business when the COVID-19 pandemic arrived in 2020. Nonetheless, the multiple challenges of the pandemic certainly exacerbated how much they struggled. These honest expressions of frustrated idealism reminded me of something that a musician friend tells aspiring guitar players who ask him for career advice. He replies, "Sure, you should become a musician. There are hundreds of dollars to be made."

Certainly, the forced shift to online spaces loosened the ties between students and particular studios. Obviously, this change is ambiguous: people can now practise and teachers can now teach in many places, both live and through recordings available on YouTube and other platforms, either for free or by subscription. For those who appreciate styles (like Ashtanga and Iyengar) that feature hands-on adjustments and long-term teacher-student relationships, the challenges are more severe.

When they could no longer rely on membership fees, many studio owners opted to merge with other studios, switch to online formats, or close. The last of several dozen YogaWorks studios in Los Angeles – where thousands of North American students and teachers were first introduced to advanced practice – shut its doors just the week before we arrived for our fieldwork in the fall of 2022. That was the most striking contraction, and many teachers and students in Los Angeles mentioned it even if they were not connected to the studio. Clearly, this closure was a symbol of a general shift that we could see in other styles and cities.

Teachers, studio owners, and entrepreneurs now face quite different market conditions than they ever have and need to be ever more involved in branding and digital curation. My own shala changed hands during the pandemic, and the new owner has opted to add other yoga and movement practices (e.g., ecstatic dance, Yin, and vinyasa yoga) to the core Ashtanga offerings (e.g., Mysore and led classes). This sort of innovation is likely to happen in other yoga communities that currently offer a single style.

The new reality facing studios raises questions for scholars interested in the economics of wellness and spiritual communities. Will often-competing lineage systems – Iyengar and Ashtanga, for example – be likely to join forces in order to prevent more closures? If that happens, how will each subcommunity reimagine its claims to authenticity? Will the move to online platforms during COVID-19 be reversed now that the pandemic appears to be mostly over? The maxim often heard in the social sciences is "Follow the money." What might we learn not just about yoga but also about our societies by examining the ways that privatized and digitally mediated wellness routines impact conviviality and traditional community life?

From Monsters to the Mundane

In every focus group and interview, we talked about the reprehensible behaviour of many of yogaland's most famous leaders. Almost all communities were affected by the scandals, and in response, a great many moved decisively to create formal or informal policies and procedures designed to clarify their position and to protect students from sexual misconduct. The spirit of these shifts certainly animated my own teacher training and is evident in hundreds of public statements made by communities across yogaland.[7] Communities such as Kripalu and Iyengar engaged in thorough internal reflections, whereas others, such as Ashtanga, conducted an analysis that seems to have been more fragmentary. As these controversies are addressed in chapter 5, I will not revisit them here.

It seems to me that studio owners and communities more generally have become experts at hunting, catching, and expelling monsters. Now that many of the major monsters have been caught or slain (or have simply retired, relocated, or died), is yogaland ready for what might be the much more difficult phase of the conversation? I doubt it. There are exceptions, but apart from the appeal of all things Tantric in yogaland (a subject that I hope to explore in another project), it seems to me that there is far less readiness or enthusiasm for talking about the deep ambiguities generated during practices (and in other social spaces) involving some measure of intimacy and vulnerability.

Teachers are normally instructed to be sure that they watch themselves and ensure that any contact with students "comes from a place of concern for the student," as one teacher put it, rather than from "sexual attraction or even appreciation." Fair enough but perhaps impossible too. A great many human interactions – whether in a yoga studio, classroom, bar, or workplace – are sexually charged to some extent, so it is exceedingly difficult for teachers and students to sequester inherently ambiguous forms of human desire. Sexual desires are just part of the human condition; the question, of course, is what one does with these feelings.

I am not – I repeat, not – suggesting that teachers and students should just do whatever they want simply because sexual feelings are common and complicated. Rather, I am suggesting that the best way to ensure that yoga spaces are in fact as free from sexual misconduct as possible is to create opportunities to talk through these ambiguities and to create the shared vocabulary and transparent processes that doing so requires. In chapter 5, I noted that many studios – especially because of the #MeToo controversies – began to ask students to place small "consent cards" near their mats to indicate whether they would welcome physical adjustments. I hand these out when I teach, and I encourage people to feel free to flip the card over if or when they change their mind. These cards represent an important step, but of course it is not a simple matter to create a culture of consent in which it is understood not only that a student needs explicitly to permit physical adjustments but also that it is necessary to reflect critically and openly on the problems associated with the complex intimacies that develop between students or between students and teachers.

However, it is hard to achieve these aims. Although we live in a society where pornography is ubiquitous, sex work is increasingly destigmatized, hook-up culture and polyamorous relationships are no longer scandalous, and there are ways to access good information about human sexuality, it is still true to say that there is a lot of unevenness in the ways that we talk about sexuality in our society.

In addition, there are a variety of opinions about what to make of the abuse. Earlier in the book, I introduced Toni, a woman I described as a jivanmukta, a significant figure in yogaland, and a fan of quantum physics. She was unflinching in her criticism of her former guru, who was part of the #MeToo controversies. However, she offered a mesmerizing account of the radically new phase into which postural yoga has moved since all the revelations surfaced. Of particular interest is her assertion that "we're coming into this time where it's about taking self-responsibility, initiating yourself into a practice, finding a teacher, finding guidance, but without that tendency to idolize and place the image of the perfect person that we're always trying to live up. And we're always falling short ... To me, it's a liberation of the teachings that no more is there this dogmatic approach to rigid guidelines around the teachings or a tightening and a gripping and a holding and an idealization."[8]

Where she and I differ in our assessments of the current moment is that she has faith that the fall of so many gurus will lead to liberation, whereas my sense is that without a serious conversation about the complex desires that arise when people are in such close contact, many more monsters will arise. Such discussions might allow us to enter the mystery so well evoked by Kai Cheng Thom in her poem "trauma is not sacred," which ends with these words:

all bodies know how to heal themselves given enough time
all demons carry a map of heaven and their scars
beneath the skin of every history of trauma

there is a love poem

waiting deep below[9]

Which yoga communities are best equipped to foster a sophisticated conversation about the scars beneath our skin, the love poems we might find
waiting deep below, the monstrous and ordinary sexualities with which we
must grapple? Will it be possible to address the erotic feelings that might
arise not just between teachers and students (the relatively easy part) but
between students (the fairly hard part)? To which bodies of research and activism do communities turn to inform their approaches (e.g., feminist research, sexual health research, and legal or human rights activism)? What
kind of impact might these discussions have on yogaland?

The Personal, the Professional, the Political

In "Bonfire Opera," the American poet Danusha Laméris captures the experience that many of us have as we try to make peace with, sense of, and
shapes with our fragile, yearning bodies. The speaker in this poem reflects
on an aging woman seemingly at peace with her own body. The speaker ad-
mires the older woman yet sees as well that this appearance of equanimity

was not the hymn of promise
but the body's bright wailing against its limits.
A bird caught in a cathedral – the way it tries
to escape by throwing itself, again and again,
against the stained glass.[10]

Most comprehensive religious, spiritual, and intellectual accounts of the
world promise to provide an escape for that bird so it is allowed to exit the
building and to fly, finally, free.

It will not remain free forever. It will get hungry, it will raise a family, its flying abilities will decline, and it will be terrorized by predators and forest fires. It will learn that buildings are containers and cages, but still, it will seek shelter among other birds.

What is this story doing here at the end of an otherwise sober account of future research directions I or others might pursue? I suppose I want to make sure to observe that a serious yoga practice resembles serious Buddhist, Christian, or Muslim practices in that these religious ways of knowing, moving, thinking, and being reflect an abiding urge to be free.

But free from what? Certainly, free from suffering caused by the psychological, social, and historical forces that agitate our minds and burden our bodies. Earlier, I mentioned the core definition of yoga offered in Patanjali's *Yoga Sutras* (1.2), translated by Iyengar as "the cessation of movements in the consciousness,"[11] or by my first asana teacher, Jack, as "the controlling, or channelizing, of the whirlpools of the mind-stuff." The benefit of a serious commitment to yoga – here I have in mind more than just asanas – is explained in the next verse (1.3), where Patanjali writes, according to Iyengar, "Then the seer dwells in his own true splendour,"[12] or as Jack put it, "Then the seer resides in their own true nature."

The challenge is that whether one is a curious critic or a devoted practitioner, modern postural yoga communities reflect the core values, aesthetics, prejudices, and ideologies of the societies in which yoga has been embedded. That should not come as a great surprise since nothing that we value – our countries, families, laws, and most mundane habits – exists in a vacuum. Yoga might promise its practitioners radical freedom, and jivanmuktas (superpeople) might make asanas look effortless, but the postures, the people, and the places in which they meet are enmeshed in a broader world of samsara (the cycle of birth, death, and rebirth) that is exceedingly difficult to escape. Difficult, but some mornings on the mat in my shala, it seems not impossible to imagine that the bird might finally find a way into the sky beyond the stained glass.

This book has been animated – perhaps haunted – by the question of how people might think dispassionately about something they love passionately. How might scholar-practitioners balance their understandable tendency to defend a liberating practice with their responsibility to provide a credible intellectual analysis of a practice? And would such a balancing act interest people who are only scholars or only practitioners? Are people fundamentally diminished or enhanced when they outgrow an innocent approach to their most deeply held values, teachers, beliefs, and practices? I cannot answer these questions definitively, but my sense is that one finds in yogaland a growing sympathy both for those who are curious about the history and composition of stained glass and for those who identify with the bird in the cathedral.

Notes

Introduction

1   Mysore is a city in the state of Karnataka in South India (population 1.2 million). It is associated with the origins of the asana-oriented styles of yoga that we see in North America.

2   Some academic readers may wince to see Sanskrit asana and philosophical terms without the diacritical marks (accents, dots, squiggles, and so forth) that normally accompany them. After seeing so many variations in the ways that these words are rendered in English, I consulted a Sanskritist in Los Angeles and decided that it would be preferable to use a standardized and unadorned spelling. In an attempt to make the reading experience as smooth as possible, I have also opted not to italicize Sanskrit words.

3   See Van der Veer and Vertovec, "Brahmanism Abroad."

4   The story of the appeal of Vivekananda is told in a variety of places. See De Michelis, "Modern Yoga: Transmission."

5   In the nineteenth and early twentieth centuries, Unitarianism was a very liberal, scholarly form of Protestantism most popular among small communities of North America's and Britain's intellectual elite. In the subsequent fifty years, it would distance itself from Christianity. By the time my mother became a minister in the 1980s, many Unitarians would know (or care) very little about their once Protestant history.

6   Concerning the influences of these Western sensibilities on yoga in India and in the West, see De Michelis, "Modern Yoga: Transmission"; Halbfass, *India and Europe*; and Lavan, *Unitarians and India*. It is worth noting that Paramahansa Yogananda, another crucial figure in the arrival of postural yoga in North America, was invited to the United States to speak at a conference featuring liberal religionists. Not only did the invitation come from the American Unitarian Association (the predecessor of the current Unitarian Universalist Association), but on his speaking tours of the United States he

also often spoke in Unitarian churches. See "Swami Yogananda Giri Speaks on 'the Inner Life,'" *Boston Globe*, 5 March 1921.

7 See Bramadat, *Church on the World's Turf*.

8 De Michelis defines this term as "those styles of yoga practice that put a lot of emphasis on *asanas* or yoga postures; in other words, the more physical or gymnastic-like type of yoga." De Michelis, *History of Modern Yoga*, 4.

9 Alter, *Yoga in Modern India*; Bryant, *Yoga Sutras of Patanjali*; De Michelis, *History of Modern Yoga*; Foxen, *Inhaling Spirit*; Jain, *Selling Yoga*; Jain, *Peace Love Yoga*; Mallinson and Singleton, *Roots of Yoga*; Miller, *Embodying Transnational Yoga*; Singleton, *Yoga Body*; White, ed., *Yoga in Practice*. See also the work emerging from the Centre of Yoga Studies, School of Oriental and African Studies, University of London (https://www.soas.ac.uk/search?search=yoga) and from the Yoga Studies Program, Loyola Marymount University, Los Angeles (https://bellarmine.lmu.edu/yoga/).

10 For more context, see McCartney, "Spiritual Bypass," 140–1: "Let us begin with describing Yogaland; which is the emic, and sometimes euphemistic, term used by many yoga practitioners and teachers to describe the global yoga community. Increasingly, Yogaland's boundaries expand beyond physical localities, and particularly, the borders of nation states, to fuel the utopian possibility of a post-national alternative … From the physical locality of a local yoga studio, Yogaland becomes a metaphor; or rather, a psychological entity that exists in the minds of those who describe their yoga tribe as being a part of something greater than the sum of its parts … Principally, Yogaland exists in the social imaginary landscape. It is a utopian inspired meta-space where life is celebrated, and various yoga-inflected lifestyles are promoted as the antithesis to, or, a distraction from, the perceived disenchantment that many people feel is a direct consequence of the hyper-routinisation of the neoliberal-inspired, late-modern, post-secular modernity. The irony is that the multibillion-dollar global yoga industry is modelled on neo-liberal ideology, which the Indian state blends with the guru-devotee relationship in the pursuit of certain ends."

11 This categorization reflects an ex post facto exercise on my part, but other examples of this genre can be found in the series of texts Writing Lives: Ethnographic and Autoethnographic Narratives, published by Routledge.

12 In formal interviews, participants first read and then signed a detailed consent form. These interviews were recorded and transcribed, whereas the informal ones were more casual and unrecorded; nonetheless, they often addressed the key project questions. We had dozens of other interactions from which we

learned a great deal about yoga and the broader culture of the cities and studios; we did not include these interactions in the tally of interviews because participants did not directly address project themes.

13 I also conducted a survey that confirmed what we learned in the interviews, which is that many (nearly 60 per cent) practise at home on their own, either with or without the guidance of pre-recorded classes on YouTube or Peloton. I should note that the survey sample is skewed toward very committed yogis (with 44 per cent of participants indicating that they practise five to seven times each week). When practising at home, practitioners nonetheless often follow the form prescribed by a lineage or style, such as Ashtanga, Iyengar, or Yin, or they may improvise their own sequences. It would have been quite invasive to watch people practise at home, so our fieldwork took place in yoga contexts where people practise in groups. Although we could not observe people practising on their own, we did get insights into their priorities and preferences through the survey. To the best of my knowledge, all of the studio-oriented students and teachers we interviewed also practised at home. In some cases, our interviews with teachers took place in their homes and often in their home-based practice spaces. The survey is available on the main website of the Centre for Studies in Religion and Society at the University of Victoria: https://www.uvic.ca/research/centres/csrs/index.php.

14 The identities of all participants in this book have been hidden by giving them pseudonyms or by altering certain elements of their life histories. Doing so was not entirely possible in the case of my own main teachers, but they have seen and approved the stories in which they appear. As well, I should note that interview and focus group subjects responded to invitations from me or heard about the project through word of mouth, colleagues in the Yoga in Theory and Practice unit at the American Academy of Religion, or promotions on posters, Facebook, or Instagram.

15 I speculate that we would find a similar dynamic at work within the ostensibly secular and often medicalized mindfulness programs that are by now ubiquitous in corporations, governments, universities, and hospitals. From reading the biographies of teachers and from interacting with them at these workshops, one would realize quickly that this or that teacher has spent months in a monastery in Thailand or California. We might also learn that a teacher can read Pali, or that a teacher has a very strong grasp of stories of the Buddha's life, or that a teacher has met the Dalai Lama, Pema Chodron, or Thich Nhat Hahn at workshops. So it turns out that these teachers' spiritual biographies are crucial features of their (secular) professional

self-presentation and self-understanding. These conventional religious discourses convey authority and authenticity to them, even though they are officially teaching people about techniques that need not be restricted to capital-R religious communities.

16 The project research assistant, an American doctoral student in the University of Victoria's Anthropology Department, joined me for five of the six visits to cities beyond Victoria, but for the second last city visit (Los Angeles), I was accompanied by the research and program coordinator of the Centre for Studies in Religion and Society. It was worthwhile to introduce a new colleague to the ethnographic process, especially since she was able to observe and inquire critically about things to which the doctoral student and I had become accustomed.

17 A synopsis of the survey's questions and main findings is available on the main website of the Centre for Studies in Religion and Society (CSRS): https://www.uvic.ca/research/centres/csrs/index.php. The survey was conducted through the Qualtrics platform and was promoted over about six months, directly and indirectly, through networks associated with the CSRS, the Yoga in Theory and Practice unit at the American Academy of Religion, the Yoga Alliance, and dozens of social media groups related to major yoga communities around North America. Because of how the survey was conducted and given the number of people who completed the survey, the 650-person sample is a "convenience sample," as opposed to a more fully representative sample. However, the sample was large enough and the geographical spread of the participants was wide enough that this resource is still valuable. To the best of my knowledge, no survey like this one has ever been undertaken.

18 Academic readers understandably expect a "literature review" in the early phases of a scholarly book. Since this book straddles a few genres, I have opted not to clutter the pages with parenthetical references. In the text itself and certainly in the endnotes and bibliography, I hope that readers will see the connections between what I am doing and the broader field of yoga studies. To provide newcomers to the field with a brief sample of the interests of these scholars, many of whom are also practitioners, I note that they encourage us to think about how "secular" public schools and prisons respond to the Indic religious symbolism and imagery of postural yoga, how the uptake of yoga in the West is used by Hindutva movements in India to propel particular policies, how the debates over what is and is not authentic yoga teach us a great deal about other tensions in our society, how sexual miscon-

duct allegations are managed by studios or lineages, and whether and why yoga tourism is popular among Western students. As well, they reflect on whether, and in what ways, during the 125 years in which yoga has been adapted in North America, it may have been democratized (with less prestige accorded to gurus and lineages), feminized (with a dramatic shift toward women practitioners and teachers), and otherwise made more available (with sometimes free classes, subsidized classes for disabled people, and classes in prisons, parks, and public schools).

19 On the Hatha Yoga Project, led by James Mallinson, see School of Oriental and African Studies, University of London, "Hatha Yoga Project."

20 Cope, *Yoga and the Quest*, 307.

21 Ibid., 308.

22 Watts, *Spiritual Turn*, 31n3.

23 The stew metaphor comes from Cope: "If you scratch the surface of the major yoga lineages that have been influential in the West, you will find a stew similar to the one with which Kripalu students were confronted – slightly different ingredients, perhaps, different tastes, different emphases, but a stew all the same." Cope, *Yoga and the Quest*, 309.

24 Ibid., 310.

25 Van der Kolk, *Body Keeps the Score*.

Chapter One

1 McCartney, "Spiritual Bypass."

2 Strauss, *Positioning Yoga*.

3 Of course, because of the COVID-19 pandemic, many students shifted their practice from studios to their homes. The experience fostered by digitally mediated classes is functionally analogous to studio settings, at least in the sense that the teachers' spaces will themselves be well curated, with attention paid to lighting, clothing, music, and so on. For home practitioners, setting aside space and meeting digitally with their teacher and yoga peers in a virtual studio similarly invite their extraction from the regular world.

4 Different schools of Indian philosophy frame the nature of reality and the ways that ignorance is sustained quite differently; these are interesting issues but well beyond the scope of this book. See Bryant, *Yoga Sutras of Patanjali*; Doniger, *Hindus*; Mallinson and Singleton, *Roots of Yoga*; and Shearer, *Story of Yoga*.

5 See Mallinson and Singleton, *Roots of Yoga*; and Bryant, *Yoga Sutras of Patanjali*.

6   Government of India, "Overview of the Department of AYUSH," 1: "Depart-
    ment of Indian Systems of Medicine and Homoeopathy (ISM&H) was created
    in March 1995 and re-named as Department of Ayurveda, Yoga & Naturo-
    pathy, Unani, Siddha and Homoeopathy (AYUSH) in November 2003 with a
    view to providing focused attention to development of Education & Research
    in Ayurveda, Yoga & Naturopathy, Unani, Siddha and Homoeopathy systems."

7   Government of India, *Common Yoga Protocol*, 2–3, 8, 9.

8   At the United Nations, Modi said, "Yoga is an invaluable gift of ancient Indian
    tradition. It embodies unity of mind and body; thought and action; restraint
    and fulfillment; harmony between man and nature and a holistic approach to
    health and well-being. Yoga is not about exercise but to discover the sense of
    oneness with ourselves, the world and Nature. By changing our lifestyle and
    creating consciousness, it can help us to deal with climate change. Let us work
    towards adopting an International Yoga Day." Government of India, *Common
    Yoga Protocol*, 1.

9   For more background on Indian demographics, see Pew Research Center,
    "Population Growth."

10 On the "weaponization" of postural yoga for the benefit of Indian nationalist
    interests, see Black, *Flexible India*; Jain, *Selling Yoga*, 168; Lal, "Politics of Yoga";
    and McCartney, "Politics beyond the Yoga Mat." In an article about the Bhara-
    tiya Janata Party's political use of postural yoga, Indian journalist Neeta Lal
    writes, "Muslim organizations in particular have objected to the Surya Na-
    maskar (a set of yoga exercises), which requires a person to bow to the Sun
    God. Points out Amina Begum, a mother of two school-going girls based in
    New Delhi, 'Islam being a monotheistic religion doesn't allow followers to
    bow before anyone except Allah. We don't like our kids following this routine
    in their schools. Surely, there are other neutral forms of exercises which can
    benefit children?'" Lal, "Politics of Yoga."

11 For a full account of this controversy, see Bramadat, "Bridge Too Far."

12 Brown, *Debating Yoga*; Nikias, "Yoga Lawsuit"; Perry, "Legal Fight."

13 Griera, "Yoga in Penitentiary Settings."

14 They do not focus on the Canadian prison system, but I suspect that their
    critique would be applicable to Canada, especially when one considers the
    massive overrepresentation of Indigenous people in the Canadian correc-
    tional system.

15 Godrej, "Neoliberal Yogi"; Jain, "Neoliberal Yoga."

16 See the websites of Yoga Gives Back (https://yogagivesback.org/); the New
    Leaf Foundation (https://newleaffoundation.com/); and Off the Mat, Into the

World (https://www.offthematintotheworld.org/). See also Yoga Alliance, "Yoga Diversity Dilemma."

17 Godrej, "Neoliberal Yogi," 775. See also Jain, "Neoliberal Yoga."

18 Marx, *Critique of Hegel's "Philosophy of Right,"* 131.

19 Strauss, *Positioning Yoga.*

20 Here, I have in mind the idea of what Benedict Anderson would call Tara's "imagined community." See Anderson, *Imagined Communities.* The point is that she is a product of a particular society – including its government, media sphere, and educational systems – that has guaranteed that she identifies mostly with people within its national borders. As a result, although Tara lives in Toronto, a massive forest fire in British Columbia is likely to concern her more than the same fire in North Carolina, even though the second fire is 3,000 kilometres closer.

21 Altglas, *From Yoga to Kabbalah.*

22 As I found in my first book, and as the project assistant reminded me, a similar thing could be said of evangelicals in North America: the Canada-US political differences certainly matter, but the broader discourse of evangelicals versus the secular (and, to use their terminology, "non-Christian") world matters more. See Bramadat, *Church on the World's Turf.*

23 Korzybski, "Non-Aristotelian System," 750.

24 For a discussion of both the political damage that can be inflicted or perpetuated through yoga and the ways that it can animate more liberative actions for individuals and groups, see Black, *Flexible India.*

25 By way of a contrast, my teacher Annie commented that the Mysore-style classes of Ashtanga yoga – in which students practice whatever portion of the asana series they have been "given" while a teacher observes their progress and intervenes with advice and adjustment when necessary – are "a hard sell." She observed that in the Mysore space, "You need to look in, and you need to look at yourself. [And people often say,] 'Well, no, I don't want to do that. I want to escape.' That's why [many] people won't do Mysore because ... [with led classes], you can zone out. I zone out when I do led classes, [so] I avoid led. But then I do [a led class], and I kind of love it because I [can] just zone out, and I just do what I'm told, and I don't have to think. And [then] you don't have to, you know, clean all the icky places, which is what Ashtanga is about."

26 Van der Kolk, *Body Keeps the Score.*

27 Sarah Strauss writes, "While Westerners may be searching for a way to escape the bonds of modern life, few of them are actually willing to go as far as renouncing the workaday world. Rather, most – like most Indians who practice

yoga – seek an oasis regime, and a way of opting out of daily life for brief periods, measured in minutes, hours, or – at the most – days." Strauss, *Positioning Yoga*, 126.

Chapter Two

1 This is what ethnographers call a composite conversation. That is, I did not record it, but I have had some variant of this discussion dozens of times in my own shala, in workshops, in other studios, in the research project that animates this book, and truth be told, throughout my whole career.

2 On yoga's role in transformative events and at festivals, Amanda Lucia writes, "It is somewhat ironic that these adamantly 'not religious' routinely invest energy in recreating the conventional religious form of the altar." Lucia, "Marking Sacred Space," 117. Also, it is worth noting that teachers and serious Ashtanga students are often encouraged to go to India to have personal contact with the lineage holder and perhaps eventually to be invited to become an authorized teacher. There are three levels: Authorized Level 1, Authorized Level 2, and Certification. To be invited by Sharath Jois to accept these roles requires a tremendous commitment to a regular practice, several long visits to Mysore, and signs of growth in one's mastery of asanas, yoga philosophy, and the related "limbs" of yoga. (Ashtanga means "eight limbs" and refers both to the system championed by Pattabhi Jois and to the broader system articulated by Patanjali and others.) This process of authorization and professionalization is temporally, financially, and physically separate from and more demanding than the Yoga Alliance's system, which uses the Registered Yoga Teacher 200-hour and 500-hour designations. The Iyengar system of training is also very rigorous, and teachers must commit to a difficult life-long system of study, tests, and scrutiny.

3 For whom is unemployment a problem – for laid-off workers, for owners, for stockholders, for government representatives, or for economists? Who is making these claims about the United States or Canada?

4 I appreciate this body of commentary tremendously. See, for example, the work of Talal Asad, Craig Martin, and Russell McCutcheon in the bibliography.

5 For example, the dramatic post-1960s shift in Quebec toward an increasingly "secular" approach to public services needs to be understood against the backdrop of centuries in which the Catholic Church exerted direct control over health care, social services, and education. However, the deep Christian roots of the society remained intact, as we saw during vitriolic public and

political debates over the past fifteen years that focused heavily on Muslim signs of public distinctiveness, such as hijabs, although the head-coverings were stand-ins for the larger communities in question. These debates brought to the surface the artificial – from the root word "to make" – nature of the distinctions made between categories such as religious and secular. The debate in Quebec produced absurdities that were apparent to people attuned to the distinctions being imagined between the religious past and the secular present and future of the province. For example, some claimed that the crucifix in the province's legislative assembly and the 30-metre-tall illuminated cross that sits on top of Mount Royal, around which the city of Montreal is built, are not religious but part of the province's cultural heritage. Similarly, the claim that public schools in the United States must be protected as "secular" often seems unproblematic, but Christian holiday schedules and festivals remain privileged.

6 Iyengar studios use the Invocation to Patanjali: "Yogena cittasya padena vacam malam sarirasya ca vaidyakena yopakarottam pravaram muninam patanjalim pranajaliranato'smi abahu purusakaram sankha cakrasi dharinam sahasra sirasam svetam pranamami patanjalim." Translation: "Let us bow before the noblest of sages Patanjali, who gave yoga for serenity and sanctity of mind, grammar for clarity and purity of speech and medicine for perfection of health. Let us prostrate before Patanjali, an incarnation of Adisesa, whose upper body has a human form, whose arms hold a conch and a disc, and who is crowned by a thousand-headed cobra." See https://iyengaryoga.org.uk/resources-2/sounds/.

7 This is the translation and punctuation found in an essay written by Sharath Jois, the current Ashtanga lineage holder. Jois, "Sharath Jois on the Essence." This authorship does not make the translation authoritative, of course. I have heard and chanted other versions at Ashtanga studios. Zoë Slatoff, a scholar of Sanskrit and a senior Ashtanga teacher, offers another translation. See Slatoff, "Sacred Sound."

8 Patanjali is honoured with invocations, statues, and shrines in most modern schools of yoga, including Iyengar yoga and Ashtanga vinyasa yoga. The yoga scholar David Gordon White writes that yoga teacher training often includes "mandatory instruction" in the *Yoga Sutras*. White calls this required instruction "curious to say the least." In his view, the text is essentially irrelevant to "yoga as it is taught and practiced today" since the *Yoga Sutra* is "nearly devoid of discussion of postures, stretching, and breathing." White, *Yoga Sutra of Patanjali*, 1.

9   The Iyengar training process is similarly, and perhaps even more, rigorous. See B.K.S. Iyengar Yoga, "How to Become."

10 Woodhead and Brown, *That Was the Church*; Heelas and Woodhead, *Spiritual Revolution*; Watts, *Spiritual Turn*.

11 The decline of many Christian organizations is what I mean here since they are the major players when it comes to large shifts in opinions about North American religion.

12 Beyer and Ramji, *Growing Up Canadian*.

13 Bramadat, O'Connell Killen, and Wilkins-LaFlamme, eds, *Religion at the Edge*.

14 This perspective was echoed by another African American teacher in Los Angeles. Kadisha said, "The African American community has not [embraced yoga] … For most [may] not necessarily have felt welcome in the yoga space. They think that's not necessarily for them … And so, for me, it's educating the community about yoga. But yoga, capital-Y, is not just the physical practice but all of the practices and more from a philosophical standpoint and recognizing, helping people recognize, like it could be spiritual. It doesn't have to be religious; it doesn't have to be Hinduism, Buddhism. If you're comfortable with Christianity, it could be in that space. It's the god within you."

15 By way of another example of the lines that get drawn between physical, religious, spiritual, and secular orientations, consider Ruth's reflection: "There is nothing religious about helping someone see themselves, whether it's, you know, increasing your proprioception [i.e., sense of your body's positioning in space] and your body awareness, whether it's learning how to control your own nervous system, using your breath. I mean, these are just physiological things that we're talking about. This isn't spiritual, but the, the process of learning about yourself is an inherently spiritual experience … My belief is that if you are an inherently spiritual person, and if you practice yoga regularly, and you breathe in and out in this way, and you move your body in this way, that spirituality will find you. I don't believe that it's my job to make you spiritual or to help you be spiritual. I don't connect spiritually with Judaism [her birth tradition]. I connect culturally with Judaism. I connect spiritually with yoga, but I don't connect religiously with yoga." John also said, "I separate religion and spirituality, though. So, to me, for [anything to] be secular doesn't mean it's not spiritual. It means it's not religious. So there's no doctrine in my classes … apart from 'Do what I say.'"

16 Smith, *Soul Searching*, 175.

17 The exception, at least for now, would be some evangelical communities that

are holding their own or growing in some cases. In addition, relative new-comer communities continue to grow rapidly, although this is almost entirely because of immigration.

18 Bramadat et al., eds, *Urban Religious Events*.

19 Black, *Flexible India*.

20 Bramadat, "Bridge Too Far."

21 "Instead of economy being embedded in social relations, social relations are embedded in the economic system." Karl Polanyi, quoted in Frerichs, "Karl Polanyi," 200.

22 Sherov-Ignatiev and Sutyrin, "Peculiarities and Rationale"; Scott, "Rise of India."

23 For more in-depth accounts of this story, see Singleton, *Yoga Body*; and De Michelis, *History of Modern Yoga*.

24 To be clear, this generalization does not capture all practitioners. Some advanced students and teachers – although not very many – have spent months or years in India and are very well acquainted with its political complexities. On the ambiguous uses and meanings of postural yoga in the Indian context – but also elsewhere in yogaland – see Black, *Flexible India*.

25 The term "hatha" usually refers to the "yoga of force," as opposed to the yoga of devotion, strictly mental effort, ritual, or spiritual grace. However, the term is used quite loosely in yogaland. Sometimes people in Ashtanga settings use the term to mean "less strenuous" or even "easy," but sometimes the term means "all yoga involving effort," which would include Ashtanga and Iyengar.

26 Rather controversial is the evidence that his system combined existing hatha yoga traditions and techniques and a variety of European forms of "physical culture," such as gymnastics, calisthenics, and military exercises. See Jain, *Selling Yoga*; Singleton, *Yoga Body*; and Mallinson and Singleton, *Roots of Yoga*.

27 Altglas, *From Yoga to Kabbalah*; Gleig, "Culture of Narcissism Revisited"; Singleton and Goldberg, eds, *Gurus of Modern Yoga*; Goldberg, *Path of Modern Yoga*.

28 Even teachers who are not oriented toward athletes and movie stars often feel that their ambitions ought to be very limited. June, a vinyasa and hot yoga teacher, said, "You know, my kind of philosophy is if you can hold a space where the student feels better when they leave, you've done your job. It doesn't matter if you talk about chakras ... If they feel better, that's what the practice is about."

29 For a fascinating combination of theology (usually meant to make insiders

better insiders) and religious studies (usually meant to help outsiders understand the lives, institutions, and cultural products of insiders), see Thatamanil, *Circling the Elephant*.

30 These terms are political in the sense that they reflect site-specific tensions between church and state, the individual and society, the individual and caste,
the economy and the individual, owners and workers, this denomination
and that denomination, enchanted and disenchanted, Western and Eastern,
and Occidental and Oriental. These are the main – but not the only – social
tensions that lead people to assume and to promote very specific (and again,
site-specific) distinctions between religion, spirituality, and secularity.

31 Foxen, *Inhaling Spirit*.

Chapter Three

1 Oliver, "Wild Geese," 347.

2 The word "trauma" is derived from the Greek word for "wound."

3 According to the Centre for Addictions and Mental Health, "Trauma is a term
used to describe the challenging emotional consequences that living through
a distressing event can have for an individual. Traumatic events can be difficult to define because the same event may be more traumatic for some people
than for others. However, traumatic events experienced early in life, such as
abuse, neglect and disrupted attachment, can often be devastating. Equally
challenging can be later life experiences that are out of one's control, such as
a serious accident, being the victim of violence, living through a natural dis-
aster or war, or sudden unexpected loss. When thoughts and memories of the
traumatic event don't go away or get worse, they may lead to posttraumatic
stress disorder (PTSD), which can seriously disrupt a person's ability to regu-
late their emotions and maintain healthy relationships." Centre for Addictions
and Mental Health, "Trauma."

4 His focus is a Buddhist response to trauma, although as Epstein notes,
"Trauma happens to everyone. Some traumas – loss, death, accidents, disease,
and abuse – are explicit; others – like the emotional deprivation of an unloved
child – are more subtle; and some, like my own feelings of estrangement,
seem to come from nowhere. But it is hard to imagine the scope of an individual life without envisioning some kind of trauma, and it is hard for most
people to know what to do about it." Epstein, *Trauma of Everyday Life*, 11.

5 Jones, "Traumatized Subjects."

6 Some people, of course, experience or witness dramatic events – a car accident, the attacks of 11 September 2001, the Second World War – and quickly

integrate these painful events into their existing idea of the world or their self. Or they alter their sense of the world or their self and move on. This is not to say that they were not disturbed, even enraged, by the events that they witnessed but only that their existing mental architecture and social support network were such that the events did not haunt them months and years in the future. Just as trauma has become what Lexi Pandell describes as "the word of the decade," there are, predictably, people such as Michael Scheeringa who are critical of how loosely the term is used. Pandell, "How Trauma"; Scheeringa, *Trouble with Trauma.*

7   Many people are exposed to van der Kolk and Maté through articles that they have written, interviews in which they are featured, and workshops that they have provided. YouTube, Facebook, Twitter/X, and their own websites provide curious people with hundreds of ways to access their work. For their respective websites, see https://www.besselvanderkolk.com/; and https://drgabor mate.com/.

8   Eva also noted, "So I have actually experienced quite a bit of trauma in my life. And well, I'll be open with you guys. My father passed away when I was twenty years old. So I had been teaching for about two years at this point. And I remember taking a class about a month after he passed away … and I hated it because yoga made me feel and I did not want to feel. And I remember going up to my mom and crying after class and saying, 'I hate this. I never want to do yoga again. I don't want to feel this – it is too many emotions. It's too raw.' And she was like, 'You know what? That's your first class back. Try it again. Just go back. See how you feel.' And I got more used to feeling as opposed to numbing."

9   See https://www.besselvanderkolk.com/resources/the-body-keeps-the-score. Psychiatrist Ruth Lanius notes, "*The Body Keeps the Score* eloquently articulates how overwhelming experiences affect the development of brain, mind, and body awareness, all of which are closely intertwined. The resulting derailments have a profound impact on the capacity for love and work. This rich integration of clinical case examples with ground-breaking scientific studies provides us with a new understanding of trauma, which inevitably leads to the exploration of novel therapeutic approaches that allow the brain to 're-wire' itself, and help traumatized people to (re)-engage in the present. This book will provide traumatized individuals with a guide to healing and permanently change how psychologists and psychiatrists think about trauma and recovery." Lanius, quoted at *The Body Keeps the Score*'s website.

10   Van der Kolk, *Body Keeps the Score*, 53.

11 In my university and elsewhere, the trauma that students bring with them – in their bodies and into our classrooms – is discussed at many faculty meetings, where we are encouraged to be aware of and to work around the ways that our course content and student-teacher interactions might "trigger" students who have been traumatized and may lead them to be unable to meet course expectations (and might in fact "retraumatize" them).

12 "Proprioception" is defined as a "sense of body positioning in space," which "is an important bodily neuromuscular sense. It falls under our 'sixth sense,' more commonly known as somatosensation." *Physiopedia*, "Proprioception."

13 On the traumatogenic, or that which generates trauma, see Lannert, "Traumatogenic Processes."

14 As van der Kolk puts it in *The Body Keeps the Score*, 97, "Traumatised people chronically feel unsafe inside their bodies: The past is alive in the form of gnawing interior discomfort."

15 Hertzog Young, "Diagnosing Climate Disorder"; Baudon and Jachens, "Scoping Review."

16 American Psychiatric Association, "Climate Change."

17 "Economist John Williamson coined the term 'Washington Consensus' in 1989, in reference to a set of ten market-oriented policies that were popular among Washington-based policy institutions, as policy prescriptions for improving economic performance in Latin American countries." Some of the key policy reforms of the Washington Consensus period of the 1980s and 1990s, which relied on structural adjustment programs, included privatization, fiscal discipline, and trade openness. These reforms were introduced by international financial institutions as conditions for the debt relief of highly indebted, economically constrained African countries. Archibong, Coulibaly, and Okonjo-Iweala, "How Have the Washington Consensus Reforms?"

18 A variant of this metaphor is found in the nineteenth-century German stories of Baron von Munchhausen, who lifts himself and his horse out of a mire when he manages to pull himself up by his own ponytail.

19 Guest, *Neoliberal Religion*.

20 Brown, *Undoing the Demos*.

21 Hari, "Opposite of Addiction." As Tamsin Jones notes, "Moreover, with both saturating and traumatizing events there is a need for a plurality of witnesses to give testimony to, or to interpret, the event over and over again. 'Bearing witness to' entails speaking but also listening and acting." Jones, "Traumatized Subjects," 157.

22 Wittich and McCartney, "Changing Face."

23 See the *Yoga Is Dead* podcast series at https://www.yogaisdeadpodcast.com/home.

24 Michael noted, "Oh yes, I have proper health insurance. Yeah, and [yet] I still don't know, like, what my copay is … If I have to have surgery, or if I'm in an accident, or if, you know, I need to take a drug that is not covered in the giant list of drugs … Yeah. Like I have no idea what I will pay, and I don't know if it's going to be mystically, magically covered like entirely, and I will pay nothing, or if a bill for $65,000 will come in the mail."

25 American readers might be interested to know that Canadian employers often offer supplemental health care plans to their employees. These plans often allow patients to have private or semi-private rooms and may pay for chiropractic care, massage therapy, travel insurance, and certain dental and pharmaceutical services, for example. These plans are not meant to cover regular direct health care costs such as visits to emergency rooms, urgent care, mental-health services, surgery, cancer care, family physician care, and hospital care, which are covered by the publicly funded Medicare system.

26 Yogis in both Los Angeles and New York clearly saw themselves as living in unique zones, with *relatively* good public health programs. Here, "relatively" is an important modifier since they compared themselves *not* to the taxpayer-funded public health care that they might receive in almost all other liberal democratic societies in the world. Rather, New Yorkers and Los Angelinos often described their cities or states as being akin to distinct countries within the United States and indicated that the health care that they received there was superior compared to what most other Americans, especially those in the southern states, received.

27 I say "almost never" because there are always (rare) exceptions. My nephew was diagnosed with a tenacious stage-four neuroblastoma when he was just over two years old. Once the Ontario medical system had exhausted the treatment options, his parents found an experimental cancer protocol underway at Memorial Sloane-Kettering Cancer Center in New York. The cost of the lengthy and difficult treatment was roughly US$300,000, which is staggering by Canadian standards, but the family found the money to cover what turned out to be life-saving treatment. Thanks to formidable parents and an appeal to the Ontario Health Insurance Program, the parents were repaid.

28 Maddeaux, "Yes, Overturning Roe v. Wade."

29 I realize I am working on the assumption that the students and teachers we interviewed all supported a woman's right to abortion services. That might not have been the case, although we certainly heard nothing from our inter-

view subjects that would come close to being support for the US Supreme Court's overturning of the original 1967 decision. It is not impossible that some of the people we met with might have been reluctant to share their views with us.

30 See Bramadat, Berger, and MacDonald, "COVID-19 Vaccine." Johns Hopkins University published death rates for all societies. As of late January 2023, the rates for the United States and Canada were 3,383 per million and 1,307 per million respectively.

31 See respectively https://yogawithadriene.com/; https://jessamynstanley.com/; and https://kinoyoga.com/.

32 Epstein, *Trauma of Everyday Life*.

33 Chutkan, *Microbiome Solution*.

34 With regard to dissociation, Philip M. Bromberg observes, "The price for this protection is to plunder future personality development of its resiliency and render it into a fiercely protected constellation of relatively unbridgeable self-states, each rigidly holding its own truth and its own reality 'on call,' ready to come 'on stage' as needed, but immune to the potentially valuable input from other aspects of self." Quoted in Epstein, *Trauma of Everyday Life*, 73. Here, Epstein also notes that "one of the consequences of this defense is that the self is depleted of emotional depth and fluidity."

35 McGuire, *Lived Religion*.

36 Jones, "Traumatized Subjects," 156. On the importance of bodily practices such as eating, singing, and breathing as means of physical and spiritual transformation in yoga communities, see Miller, *Embodying Transnational Yoga*. See also Lucia, "Marking Sacred Space," 115, where she notes that Courtney Bender says of her "new metaphysicals" that "the physical and fleshy body can be a 'container,' but it is also a channel, conduit, or 'switch.' Meditation, yoga, Reiki, acupuncture, and a variety of other activities provided ways to find and maintain physical bodies that were open, aligned, or relaxed, and therein properly attuned to the energies that simultaneously coursed through them and constituted them." See Bender, *New Metaphysicals*, 93. Readers might also be interested in Sarah Strauss's reflections on Sivananda yoga as an illustration of embodied knowledge. Strauss, *Positioning Yoga*.

37 A few of the senior yoga teachers I met who have significant training in health sciences said that they wished that other yoga teachers would speak more modestly about the health benefits of yoga, which, in the opinions of the senior teachers, are not yet entirely settled. However, there are promising developments. The Kaivalyadhama Institute in Lonavala in Western India

continues to be the South Asian hub of scientific research on yoga. See the institute's website at https://kdham.com/. See also the *Journal of Applied Yoga Studies* at https://digitalcommons.lmu.edu/jays/, which is moored in the Yoga Studies program at Loyola Marymount University in Los Angeles.

38   For the definition of "proprioception," see note 13.

39   "Interoception" is defined narrowly as "the awareness of internal bodily signals such as heartbeat, breath, thirst, hunger, desire and pain, but the definition has evolved over decades to become more comprehensive. The *broad* definition goes beyond pure body sensation representations and includes how individuals interpret and react to these sensations." Khoury, Lutz, Schuman-Olivier, "Interoception in Psychiatric Disorders," 251.

40   Lessing, "Prisons We Choose."

41   Mallinson and Singleton, *Roots of Yoga*; Sarbacker, *Tracing the Path*; White, ed., *Yoga in Practice*.

42   Here, I should note the influence of a "lived religion" perspective on my own thinking. See McGuire, *Lived Religion*. Proponents of this critical perspective maintain that the most interesting parts of any religious community or set of claims is not its formal, doctrinal, systematic aspects, which are usually propounded by, and of interest to, a very small minority of elite males. These formal articulations of what any religion is – its theologies, dogmas, epistemologies, textual canons, ritual rules, ecclesiological structures, impressive architectural expressions, and elaborately articulated pantheons – are important objects of study for scholars, but they have received an inordinate amount of attention over the past 150 years. What has received relatively short shrift in the study of religion are the sometimes counterintuitive ways that people actually use the symbols, ideas, texts, textiles, foods, and clothing that they were given at birth. Proponents of the lived religion approach encourage students and scholars to set aside an interest in systematic theologies, formal rules, and official or canonical texts. Instead, commentators are encouraged to attend to everyday practices of ordinary people – especially women and others of nonelite status who have not enjoyed the spotlight for centuries. Moreover, a lived religion approach allows us to see the way that religion is never sui generis, or uniquely ahistorical, but a reflection of the efforts of individuals who are operating under the influence of powerful social forces that they rarely see clearly.

43   There is a massive theological and philosophical literature on these terms within Samkhya philosophy, which is the school often associated with Patanjalian yoga. This tension is well beyond the scope of this book, but readers

interested in learning about these concepts can consult Bryant, *Yoga Sutras of Patanjali*; or Sarbacker, *Tracing the Path*.

44 As I do not read Sanskrit, I am agnostic about this rendering of the term "yoga." It may be a slight misunderstanding of the original term yuj, which appears to mean something closer to "yoke," akin to what Anya Foxen and Christa Kuberry describe as the "rigging" that one might find on a chariot or sailboat. Foxen and Kuberry, *Is This Yoga?* 4, 6. Nonetheless, the reading of the term is itself instructive and speaks to the tendency of insiders to render such concepts in ways that suit their (necessarily mixed) interests.

45 Epstein, *Trauma of Everyday Life*.

46 As Jones puts it, "The aspect of trauma theory I find most helpful ... is the fact that it refuses, in a forceful way, the temptation to identify a quick fix ... And for those who do endure, recovery is a very long, nonlinear, complicated, and painful journey in which what is 'recovered' is certainly not what had been there before; there is no going back to a pristine Eden." Jones, "Traumatized Subjects," 160.

47 Although Lincoln's interest was mainly in *societies* that could be understood in these ways, it is worthwhile to extend the metaphor so as to capture differences in the ways that *individuals* understand themselves and their religious and spiritual practices. See Lincoln, *Holy Terrors*.

Chapter Four

1 The clothing will reflect the yoga style. At a hot (or Bikram) yoga studio, people wear very little clothing given that the pre-heated room temperature is roughly 36 to 40 degrees Celsius (97 to 105 degrees Fahrenheit); at an Iyengar studio, people often dress in loose pants and long sleeve shirts or modest T-shirts; and at an Ashtanga studio, people wear fashions that range between these two poles.

2 The Latin word *genius*, from *gignere* (to beget) – which also refers to the spirit present at one's birth – is the basis for the Arabic word *jinn*, often translated as "genie." It is crucial to police the tendency to project and fantasize about the uniqueness of any individual. We are all products of histories, societies, families, genetics, social classes, empires, and other factors for which we have no responsibility. Nevertheless, I also do not doubt the experience that many of us have had when in the actual or mediated presence of certain preternaturally gifted people.

3 Wittich and McCartney, "Changing Face."

4 The word "jivanmukta" also refers to an official brand or denomination of

yoga created in the 1980s by New Yorkers Sharron Gan and David Life. See
https://jivamuktiyoga.com/teachers-global/david-life/. In this chapter, I do
not address this brand, although it has been well covered by others. See Jain,
Selling Yoga.

5   I am interested in the ways that these aesthetic norms are adopted in yogaland
and in their impact on practitioners, especially the women who are the overwhelming majority in yogaland and therefore the ones who are the main
subjects and targets of the images that carry these often exclusive norms.
However, the situation is ambiguous. Most teachers and advanced students
sincerely affirm the value and appeal of all bodies, yet serious practice makes
most bodies more conventionally fit, a fact that many practitioners appreciate
even while often hearing that this outcome should not be the goal – but
rather an incidental by-product – of a serious practice. Nonetheless, the images that dominate the real and virtual neighbourhoods of yogaland do represent what, for many of us, would be an unattainable standard of beauty and
physical prowess as well as body types that closely resemble the jivanmuktas
I sketch in this chapter. As I mention in the book's afterword, I am also interested in the ways that sexual relations, imagery, and energies are imagined
and managed in yogaland. I plan to pursue these linked issues in future research, but for now, suffice it to say that the narrowness of yogaland's aesthetic norms is demonstrable, complicated, and worthy of serious critical
attention.

6   On this issue, see the work of critical theorists such as Russell McCutcheon.

7   In addition to the survey conducted for this project, the Pacific Northwest
Social Survey was an important part of a major project on religion and
spirituality (including yoga) in the Pacific Northwest. Bramadat et al., eds,
Religion at the Edge. See also Wittich and McCartney, "Changing Face"; and
Yoga Alliance, *Yoga in the World.*

8   I have in mind not just the physiques of the students relative to others in the
city where the studio is located but especially also the physiques of those who
make it onto the websites and to the front of the classes.

9   Stringfellow, "Politics of Yoga Pants"; Creel, "How Much?"

10 In fairness to the yoga industry, an "all-inclusive" month at most yoga studios
costs about $130 to $150 (with some variation between cities), which is
roughly the same amount as most comprehensive gym memberships, a single
session with a psychotherapist, one or two sessions with a chiropractor, one
or two date nights each month (assuming the cost of dinner plus a movie), or
two sessions with a personal trainer. I do practise more than most people, but

given that I go to the studio six times each week, I spend about $4 per hour. In fact, one could say that my practice saves me the cost of monthly or weekly visits with a therapist, chiropractor, and personal trainer, the cumulative cost of which would be much higher than what I currently pay. There is real merit in the critique of the cost of drop-in asana classes, which cost roughly $20 to $30 per class (or roughly five times what I spend per hour); but most studios offer a variety of payment options beyond the drop-in fee.

11   See Vanzee Taylor, dir., *I am Maris*; and Neumark-Sztainer et al., "Yoga and Pilates," which considers a correlation between disordered eating habits and an attraction to yoga and Pilates.

12   For a reflection on how yoga – especially Iyengar yoga – addressed one student's depression and eating disorders, see Kadetsky, *First There Is a Mountain*.

13   See Gaudiani, *Sick Enough*; and Wolf, *Beauty Myth*.

14   For background, see Lucia, *White Utopias*.

15   See respectively https://jessamynstanley.com/; and https://larugayoga.com/.

16   In some sense, I was both entirely in my element because it was a yoga studio and entirely out of my element because the studio was clearly meant for mostly African American students. For most of my life, I have passed as white within my personal and professional spheres. One of the Canadian teachers we met is Métis (with entangled Indigenous and French roots), and she said that passing as white is her superpower. This made perfect sense to me. In my youth, this power opened many doors and only failed me when my deep brown father walked into the room or answered the phone and spoke with a rich Trinidadian accent. This dissonance between how I was perceived and the truth of my heritage prompted confusion among my young friends that made me keenly aware that I was, or at least would always feel myself to be, an imposter. When I found myself in that Brooklyn studio, I realized that I was once again passing for white, but this time I also felt excluded from the form of nonwhiteness emphasized in this setting. This experience was peculiar since, after all, these African American students and teachers were engaged in Indic bodily and speech practices that were more – albeit quite distantly – mine than theirs, so to speak. These scenarios underline how artificial it is to claim ownership of these ideas and practices.

17   When I raised the question of cultural appropriation with the African American teachers I interviewed, four of them observed that they did not feel that they might be culturally appropriating yoga. When I asked why, they observed that the actual origins of yoga are in Africa. In particular, these teachers be-

lieve that yoga originated in Egypt. These teachers said that this form, called Kemetic Yoga, is evidenced in the hieroglyphics found in temples and pyramids. See McCartney, "India's Battle."

18 I should note that there is a debate about the ways that we should divide the *Yoga Sutras*. I am using the numbering system employed by Vivekananda and Swami Satchidananda Saraswati. As well, there is quite a lot of variety in the ways that people translate and interpret the *Yoga Sutras*. Some translations would not include all of these powers. The examples that I provide here are useful, if also playful, entry points into a conversation about why virtually no one we met brought up any special powers.

19 The text is a sequence of 196 compact philosophical assertions, followed by additional extrapolations, some as old as the sutras and some relatively recent, that resemble a midrash (or reflection on a biblical text or Talmud) in the Jewish textual tradition.

20 These practices have a long history in South Asia. See Mallinson and Singleton, *Roots of Yoga*; White, ed., *Yoga in Practice*; White, *Yoga Sutra of Patanjali*; and Sarbacker, *Tracing the Path*.

21 Bryant, *Yoga Sutras of Patanjali*, 368. Also, he notes, "The term *siddhi*, perfection or power, which occurs only four times in the *sūtras*, is used here to mean the supernormal powers. For a *yogī*, the powers noted in the previous *sūtra* hinder the cultivation of *samādhi*, since they entice the mind back out into the realm of *prakṛiti* ... and thus are obstacles, *upasargāh*, to the attainment of *samādhi*" (367).

22 Translation by Vivekananda at https://yogasutrastudy.info/yoga-sutra-translations/ysp-sutras3-21-3-40/.

23 Iyengar, *Light on the Yoga Sutras*, 219.

24 I suspect – although this is just a speculation – that the people I met in my travels clearly did not want to delve very deeply into these powers either because they were a little embarrassed by the matter-of-fact way that Patanjali introduces them or because they worried that they were not knowledgeable enough to talk about the deeper esoteric dimensions of the siddhis. In this sense, these sutras are not unlike the *Book of Daniel* in the Hebrew Bible and the *Book of Revelation* in the New Testament. Both texts are also fairly "trippy," to quote a yoga student referring to the fantastical aspects of these two texts and of the third pada of the *Yoga Sutras*.

25 Mallinson and Singleton, *Roots of Yoga*.

26 According to Yogananda, with Kriya Yoga, "the yogi is able to lessen or prevent the decay of tissues. The advanced yogi transmutes his cells into energy.

Elijah, Jesus, Kabir and other prophets were past masters in the use of *Kriya* or a similar technique, by which they caused their bodies to materialize and dematerialize at will." Yogananda, *Autobiography of a Yogi*, 263.

27 Often associated with both demanding physical and esoteric aspects of yoga (and with the *Hatha Yoga Pradipika* itself) are the Nath Yogis, an important community of renunciants and householders with a long history of developing special physical and spiritual powers for use in worldly endeavours. The Nath have long had a strong symbolic function within South Asian society, and indeed they continue to influence the ways that we imagine the conduct of committed Indian yogis, who are often portrayed as covering themselves in ash, carrying a staff, and wearing minimal clothing. Bouillier, *Monastic Wanderers*; Mallinson and Singleton, *Roots of Yoga*; White, *Sinister Yogis*.

28 On the training offered by Kia Miller in Rishikesh, see https://www.kiamiller.com/events/. See also My Spiritual India Tours, a company led by a yoga teacher based in New Zealand, at https://www.myspiritualindiatours.com/.

29 Comment by former Canadian ambassador James George in a television documentary about Trungpa Rinpoche's community in Nova Scotia. Cherniak, dir., "Nirvana in Nova Scotia."

30 There are, of course, dozens of other powerfully charismatic and famous Indian yogis who rarely appear in Western yoga discourse. Baba Ramdev (see Jain, *Selling Yoga*), for example, is hardly discussed at all in North American yogaland, although he is a major player in the Indian yoga, political, and business scenes. T.K.V. Desikachar is Krishnamacharya's son but is also not very well known in Western circles because of his more reserved approach to his teaching and lineage. The authority of both Sharath Jois and Geeta Iyengar combines traditional and charismatic forms since they are inheritors of a grandfather's (Jois) or a father's (Iyengar) yoga lineage. Both are also treated as though they possess charismatic gifts of their own.

31 For accounts of the recreation of yoga in the West, see Jain, *Selling Yoga*; Jain, *Peace Love Yoga*; Singleton, *Yoga Body*; and Syman, *Subtle Body*.

32 See respectively, Foxen, *Biography of a Yogi*; and Lore, *Hell-Bent*.

33 Foxen, *Biography of a Yogi*; Foxen, *Inhaling Spirit*; Singleton and Goldberg, eds, *Gurus of Modern Yoga*.

34 In this sense, one might say that quantum physics is often a classic "skyhook" for nonscientists in need of a scientific-sounding theory to explain something deeply implausible and for which one lacks basic evidence.

35 Another teacher in New York noted, "I never really went beyond high school

physics. But I really like listening to these geeky people talk about quarks and string theory and all these weird things that are vibrating on the inside. And I feel like they're vibrating in us. And so the vibrational breathing of yoga really resonates with me. You know, so thinking about the vibrations inside of me, and then there's vibrations outside there, and that we're creating this interference pattern of like new vibration, and then it gets very hippy. You know what I mean?"

36 See Ward and Voas, "Emergence of Conspirituality"; and Greenspan and Landsverk, "How QAnon Infiltrated."

37 On this list, one would find stars such as Eddie Stern, Kia Miller, Seane Corn, Kino MacGregor, Rachel Brathen, Richard Freeman, Noah Mazé, David Robson, Laruga Glaser, Dharma Mittra, Shiva Rea, David Swenson, Tim Miller, Dylan Werner, Mark Robberds, Deepika Mehta, and Gurmukh Kaur Khalsa. This list could be several times longer; in chapter 5, I discuss why people such as Rodney Yee, Bikram Choudhury, David Life, and John Friend are not on this partial list. One of the most massive figures in the digital yoga space is Adriene Mishler, with about 13 million YouTube subscribers. Her girl-next-door self-presentation may be the source of her tremendous popularity, and it would be interesting to consider in a future study whether she might be considered a jivanmukta by her fans.

38 This line of research echoes what we learn from what is sometimes called the "critical religion" approach or school, as seen in the work of Russell McCutcheon, for example.

39 Andrea Jain similarly argues that no one should be surprised that postural yoga took the shape that it did in North America since it has always been reconfigured by its standard-bearers to reflect (and perhaps critique) the dominant ideologies of the times and places in which it is situated. Jain, *Selling Yoga*.

40 Putnam, *Bowling Alone*.

41 Here, I have in mind the work of Liz Bucar, Anya Foxen, Andrea Jain, Christa Kuberry, Amanda Lucia, Christopher Jain Miller, Mark Singleton, David Gordon White, Theodora Wildcroft, and others who appear in the bibliography.

Chapter Five

1 See Daly, "Fake Animal News"; and Macdonald, "Animals Are Rewilding."

2 McGowan and Bambra, "COVID-19 Mortality."

3 Scientific debate about this connection is easily accessible online, but see Broad, *Science of Yoga*; and Stern, *One Simple Thing*.

4   For an example of the latter, see *Yoga Mimamsa*, the well-established journal of the Kaivalyadhama Institute, founded in 1924 by Swami Kuvalayananda. See, especially, the work of the Scientific Research Department, founded the same year. The institute's website is at https://kdham.com/about-kaivalyadhama/. See also Broad, *Science of Yoga*.

5   As well, there are several online courses and free lectures offered to practitioners who want to learn Sanskrit, improve their understanding of the *Bhagavad Gita* or the *Yoga Sutras*, or learn about the history of Tantrism, among other topics. The best example of such course work is the curriculum offered by the Yogic Studies group, organized by Seth Powell. The group's website is at https://www.yogicstudies.com/.

6   This story is generally consistent with the core insights of the lived-religion perspective. At the risk of oversimplifying, we can summarize this perspective as the stance of people engaged in religious and spiritual practices who are generally uninterested – which is not to say hostile to but literally not interested – in metaphysics and systematic theologies. I am sure that aeronautical engineering is intrinsically interesting, but when I fly, I do not think much about the plane's rivets, the Bernoulli effect, or the schematics of internal combustion engines.

7   Kale and Novetzke, "Cultural Politics of Yoga," 219.

8   On the notion of authorizing discourses, see McCutcheon, "Default of Critical Intelligence?"; on plausibility structures, see Berger and Luckmann, *Social Construction of Reality*.

9   The well-known 200-hour teacher-training curricula endorsed by the Yoga Alliance includes 100 hours of training to deal with issues closely related to the Indian origins of yoga. According to the Yoga Alliance, topics in this category "could include, but are not limited to: asanas, pranayamas, kriyas [practices to detoxify the body], chanting, mantra, meditation and other traditional yoga techniques." The Yoga Alliance also mandates that 30 of the 200 hours should deal directly with "yoga philosophy," noting that "topics in this category could include, but are not limited to: The study of yoga philosophies and traditional texts (such as the Yoga Sutras, Hatha Yoga Pradipika or Bhagavad Gita); Yoga lifestyle, such as the precept of non-violence (ahimsa), and the concepts of dharma and karma; Ethics for yoga teachers, such as those involving teacher-student relationships and community; Understanding the value of teaching yoga as a service and being of service to others through yoga (seva)." Yoga Alliance, "RYS 200 Standards." There are training programs not endorsed by the Yoga Alliance. People working in the Iyengar and Ash-

tanga orbits, for example, go through a much longer training period in North America and usually India. Both include training in Indian philosophy. Nevertheless, outside of the smaller lineage-oriented communities, certification by the Yoga Alliance clearly matters a great deal, and teachers interested in a career in yoga will generally pursue this certification.

10 This vignette occurred in a Mysore class, in which students work through an established series at their own pace, with teachers moving through the room to help students one-on-one.

11 This use of the ambiguous term "vinyasa" is somewhat misleading. It is usually translated narrowly as "to place in a special way" and, more broadly, as "to pair breath with movement." Nonetheless, it is very common in Ashtanga spaces for a teacher to say "do a vinyasa" or "take a vinyasa," which usually refers to some version of the transition that I have described.

12 Wallace, *Infinite Jest*, 203.

13 I should note that although I have experienced and observed this curt style in many places, it seems to me that it is far more common in Iyengar and Ashtanga sites than in the other, newer, forms. I should also observe that both before class and the moment that the class is over, one encounters the normal range of personae: teachers can be warm, distant, garrulous, tender, encouraging, quiet, flirty, distracted, boisterous, reverential, or matter-of-fact.

14 Vishuddhi Films, "Yogacharya BKS Iyengar's Unique Revelations."

15 Singleton, *Yoga Body*; Jain, *Selling Yoga*.

16 Kale and Novetzke, "Cultural Politics of Yoga," 222.

17 In addition, I suspect that it would have come as a surprise to most yogis in South Asian history – although I cannot know if the surprise would have been welcomed – that eventually women would far outnumber men among North American practitioners.

18 See also Kadetsky, *First There Is a Mountain*.

19 Marianne, a senior teacher in Winnipeg, put it bluntly, "I've more or less reconciled [myself] with the fact that I teach a form and present a form of yoga that has North American roots. It's not Indian." On the wall beside us, there was a poster, often seen on the walls of yoga studios, that featured dozens of small photographs of an Indian man – in this case, Pattabhi Jois – demonstrating the Ashtanga primary series asanas, with their names in Sanskrit underneath. "But then there's that," I said as I gestured to the poster. Marianne looked over my shoulder at what I was pointing at and laughed. "Right, I get it. Totally. And it's very complicated. And nuanced. And you can't necessarily draw a line in the sand and be like, and now [the yoga I teach and

practise here] is North American! ... And I don't care to try to reverse the passing of time and try to make that become more authentic to India. Heavy air quotes. Because it's not [Indian]. It's a North American form."

20 Burke, *Unbound*; Lukose, "Decolonizing Feminism."

21 Lifestyle Desk, "International Yoga Day"; YJ Editors, "Kausthub Desikachar."

22 It is important to note that as with the broader phenomenon, the alleged or confirmed misconduct in yogaland ranged widely, taking forms that included infidelity to one's wife and subsequent marriage to one's student(s), grooming students, sexual activity with students despite one's pledged celibacy, and rape.

23 For a broader consideration of these issues, see the work emerging from the Religion and Sexual Abuse Project, led by Amanda Lucia, at https://www.religionandsexualabuseproject.org/. See also Lucia, "Guru Sex"; Remski, "Yoga's Culture"; and the *Spiritual Abuse in Modern Yoga* podcast course hosted by Amelia Wood in association with the School of Oriental and African Studies, University of London, at https://yso.soas.ac.uk/product/spiritual-abuse-in-modern-yoga/.

24 The Yoga Alliance does not describe itself as a regulatory body; nor does it have the ability to close any studio or to prevent anyone from teaching. Instead, on its website, it calls itself "the largest nonprofit member association representing the global yoga community." Yoga Alliance, "About Us." That is a modest self-definition for the professional association that provides the most widely recognizable certification for the very lucrative teacher-training programs that virtually all teachers feel obligated to pursue. An affiliation with the Yoga Alliance lends an air of credibility to studios and teachers. Unfortunately, the Yoga Alliance has tremendous power that has yet to be analyzed fully, as far as I am aware. For its statement on sexual misconduct, see Yoga Alliance, "Sexual Misconduct Policy." See also Yoga Journal Staff, "#TimesUp."

25 In addition, however, I should note two other prominent controversies. Within the Iyengar community, concerns were expressed about the founder's harsh physical treatment of his students (e.g., yelling and slapping, some of which has been captured on video). For a gripping literary nonfiction account, see Kadetsky, *First There Is a Mountain*. Sexual misconduct allegations were also made against one of his trusted senior teachers, the charismatic Manouso Manos. IYNAUS Board of Directors, "MM Investigative Report." The community launched a full investigation, which marginalized Manos, even though he continues to teach "in the tradition of B.K.S. Iyengar," as stated on

his website at https://www.manouso.com/. See also Singleton and Goldberg, eds, *Gurus of Modern Yoga*; and esp. Jain, "Muktananda."

26 Wallace, "Bikram Feels the Heat."

27 Schettler, "He Faced Allegations"; Griswold, "Yoga Reconsiders."

28 Orner, dir., *Bikram*.

29 See Schettler, "He Faced Allegations." When he decided to offer a workshop – entitled "Boss Is Back" – in Vancouver in the spring of 2023, the plan was met with immediate and voluminous resistance and was cancelled a few weeks after it was announced.

30 Medin, dir., *Mysore Magic*.

31 At the end of the film, the current lineage holder, or parampara, Sharath Jois, says of his grandfather and of his own status within the community, "I feel him [Pattabhi Jois]. I feel that he's there, looking [at] what I'm doing ... I don't consider myself as a guru. Some people, they believe [in] me as a guru, some people they don't believe [in] me as a guru. The people who believe [in] me as a guru, I'm a guru, [those who do not] believe [in] me as a guru, I'm not a guru for them. So I don't consider myself as a guru ... *[long pause]*. [A] guru never says that 'I am [a] guru' ... *[long pause]*. I will be always a student."

32 Rain, "Yoga Guru Pattabhi Jois."

33 For additional perspectives on this story, see Griswold, "Yoga Reconsiders."

34 On this issue, see Karen Rain's blog at https://karenrainashtangayogaand metoo.wordpress.com/. For Gregor Maehle's reflections, see his website at https://8limbs.com/about/gregor-maehle/; and Maehle, "My Initial Response."

35 Other teachers tried to set this misconduct within the context of moral complexity; he was a multifaceted "diamond" of a person, one teacher argued. For an example of this approach, see the response from well-known teacher John Scott in his article "My Yoga Teacher." See also Karen Rain's response to Scott's approach in Maehle, "Response to John Scott's View."

36 See Grigoriadis, "Karma Crash." Friend has reinvented himself and introduced a form of yoga called Bowspring, also known as Sridaiva, based on his repudiation of the more linear approach used by others (and previously by him). His approach focuses on the fascia connective tissue in the body. Anusara itself has also been, as it were, reborn to become another form of hatha yoga but without the involvement of Friend. See the website of the Anusara School of Hatha Yoga at https://www.anusarayoga.com/.

37 These two levels of recognition and permission may be granted (and rescinded) only by the lineage holder (now Sharath Jois). The comprehensive

costs of this training are somewhat difficult to determine. Some senior teachers I consulted were reluctant to disclose the costs or indicated that their costs might have been specific to their situation or to when they visited. However, one person familiar with the system indicated that those "offered" authorization are then required to pay US$1,000 to US$1,500 plus the expenses of three trips to Mysore and six months of training; those "offered" certification are required to pay US$3,500 plus the expenses of about ten trips to Mysore and many additional months of training. All travel and accommodation costs are the responsibility of the aspiring teacher; in addition, they pay US$700 per month for the training itself. People on the official list – overseen by Jois – may be removed for a number of reasons, one of which is that authorized and certified teachers are not allowed to describe workshops or mentoring in their own shalas as official Ashtanga teacher training since students may learn to be official Ashtanga teachers only in Mysore. That is why my own teacher training workshop would be considered problematic if not for the fact that my studio owner is not authorized (and so has nothing to lose) and if not for the fact that it is called a "200-hour vinyasa foundations" program, even though it is clearly conveying the Ashtanga system. Around the world, people (like me) do teach Ashtanga yoga without being authorized or certified by Jois in India, but it is clear that the official forms of recognition – authorization and certification – convey considerable prestige and help teachers to market themselves. See Sharath Yoga Centre, "Authorisation." The Iyengar system is also expensive, highly stratified, and very demanding of its teachers. The Iyengar organization is still hierarchical, time-consuming, expensive, and complicated, but it seems to me that it is less dependent on the impressions of a single person. See B.K.S. Iyengar Yoga, "How to Become."

38 For a sympathetic account of Sivananda's community, written over a decade before these scandals became public, see Strauss, *Positioning Yoga*. For a critical account of sexual misconduct in yogaland, see Lucia, "Guru Sex"; Remski, "Shielded for Decades"; Remski, "How a #MeToo Facebook Post"; and Project Satya's three interim "Investigation Reports," dated June, August, and November 2020, at http://www.projectsatya.org/satya-investigation-reports/. For the response of Sivananda's board of directors to Salter, see Sivananda, "Statement by the Board of Directors," posted on the Sivananda website, where Vishnudevananda's image is still prominently featured.

39 Salter's allegations and the mounting evidence in the case are part of the public record, and the identity and location of the practitioner I mention below

are shielded. Moreover, this representative does not say anything especially scandalous. So I believe that it is appropriate to share this story.

40 "Guru" can be used and translated loosely, as teacher, mentor, or leader, although its etymology is sometimes traced to the Sanskrit word for "weighty" or "grave" or to the words for "darkness" and "remover." Any word with the suffix "ji" is an honorific. In my fieldwork, people used the word guruji to refer to B.K.S. Iyengar, Pattabhi Jois, Sharath Jois, Bikram Choudhury, Dharma Mittra, Yogananda, Sivananda, Sadhguru, and Amrit Desai. The prefix "Sri" or "Shri" is also an honorific. "Parampara" is a term referring to an uninterrupted chain of teachings and teachers; it means literally "one following another." The term conveys the claim that the person in question is carrying on a tradition; it has been used to refer to many yoga masters throughout history, including Sivananda, Jois, and Iyengar, but it is currently associated with – indeed, many use the term as a kind of prefix and honorific for – Sharath Jois, known as the parampara of Ashtanga yoga. The term "boss" is derived from a Dutch word meaning "master"; Bikram is often associated with the term. Indeed, the poster used for his ill-fated plans to run a yoga workshop in Vancouver in 2023 used "Boss Is Back" in its banner. I have also heard it used informally in conjunction with Sharath Jois and Iyengar. The word "swami," derived from Sanskrit words meaning "master" or "prince," is rarely used in contemporary North American circles. It was associated with figures of the nineteenth and early twentieth centuries such as Vivekananda, as well as with the guru of Yogananda, Swami Yukteswar. In chapter 4, I outlined the ways that the terms "siddha" (perfected being) and "jivanmukta" (superperson) are used to refer to people with extraordinary spiritual gifts.

41 Quoted in Griswold, "Yoga Reconsiders." This article, which was circulated widely at the peak of the scandals, captures quite well the key issues that I want to address. Writing in the *New Yorker Magazine* in 2019, Eliza Griswold stated, "Jois's abuses remained hidden for so long in part because of his overwhelming authority as a guru, which may reflect a larger problem within the culture of yoga. In traditional yogic practice, a guru is a mediator – a translator of sorts – through whom a set of teachings is passed down. Devotion to the guru is meant to symbolize devotion to the teachings, not to the man. But in the Western context gurus become rock stars, and students compete to curry favor with them. This gives gurus significant influence over their students, which is sometimes misused. 'I had this idea in me that the guru was supposed to be this all-encompassing everything,' [Ashtanga teacher and

former Jois student Eddie] Stern said. 'I, along with other people, superimposed these mythologies on top of a human being … It was a misunderstanding of what the relationship was supposed to be.'"

42 Space does not permit me to delve into the fascinating story of Yogi Bhajan, the anchor of the Kundalini Yoga movement and founder of the 3HO organization. In a magazine article on this story, Stacie Stukin quotes Philip Deslippe, a historian who specializes in Yogi Bhajan: "'I think the scandals that are coming out will leave his name and his legacy as toxic,' says Deslippe, who taught Kundalini yoga for a decade before he began scrutinizing Bhajan through an academic lens. 'He will be remembered like a Harvey Weinstein or a Jerry Sandusky of yoga, and I believe his teachings will be tainted in a way that will make it very hard to rebrand or salvage them.'" Stukin, "Yogi Bhajan Turned."

43 Gleig and Williamson, eds, *Homegrown Gurus*; Singleton and Goldberg, eds, *Gurus of Modern Yoga*. It is worth noting that since he was interviewed for the *New Yorker Magazine* piece by Eliza Griswold, Stern has stepped away from Ashtanga yoga. Griswold, "Yoga Reconsiders."

44 Matthew Remski writes, "As the #MeToo movement hits the yoga scene, women are coming forward on social media, forcing crucial questions into the spotlight that the entire industry must now confront: Is the yoga studio consistently the healing space it is advertised to be? Or has it engendered a culture in which spiritual surrender can be conflated with physical submission? Above all, practitioners must now ask how a culture with such a robust history of abuse has also been marketed as a path to bodily autonomy, spiritual awakening, and a cure-all for both mental and physical ailments." Remski, "Yoga's Culture." See also, Strauss, *Positioning Yoga*, a 2005 ethnography on Sivananda that was published before these controversies erupted due to the #MeToo movement and that also deals with issues related to yoga and health.

45 Shaw, "'Tool to Help Me.'"

46 Although the time-tested (yet also evolving) Ashtanga asanas and the respectful hands-on adjustments that I have received over the years still seem right for me, I am interested in what is sometimes called "post-lineage yoga." Wildcroft, *Post-lineage Yoga*, 5, defines post-lineage yoga as forms that appeal to practitioners "looking outside of … early sources of inspiration to determine what for them, is labelled yoga … [These practitioners] are radically altering the systems of transmission and authority that have previously been thought to define the boundaries of transnational yoga."

47 Said, *Orientalism*; Asad, *Genealogies of Religion*.

48 Kale and Novetzke, "Cultural Politics of Yoga," 211.

49 Krishnamacharya, *Yoga Makaranda*, 30.

50 Gandhi and Wolff, "Yoga and the Roots"; Jain, "Fox News Controversy." The Take Back Yoga campaign seems to have been initiated by an exchange between Aseem Shukla and Deepak Chopra on the *On Faith* blog associated with the *Washington Post*. See Vitello, "Hindu Group Stirs Debate." As this debate made clear, Shukla feels that yoga is fundamentally "Hindu" rather than simply "Indian." See also Bucar, *Stealing My Religion*; Lau, "Re-Orientalism"; and Lau and Mendes, *Re-Orientalism*.

51 For the *Yoga Is Dead* podcast, see https://www.yogaisdeadpodcast.com/home.

52 "It is thus a small proportion of India's population in terms of caste and class that make up the majority of the population of Indian Americans, which also supplies the key voice in the critique of yoga as cultural appropriation." See Kale and Novetzke, "Cultural Politics of Yoga," 221.

53 Singleton, *Yoga Body*; Jain, *Selling Yoga*.

54 Wildcroft, *Post-lineage Yoga*, 5. See also Sarbacker, *Tracing the Path*; and Shearer, *Story of Yoga*.

55 Of course, Cathy is a pseudonym, but her actual name echoed the current cultural biases against the "Karen" archetype of a privileged white woman.

56 Kale and Novetzke, "Cultural Politics of Yoga," 218.

57 The results were similar when I asked people about the importance of their teachers' and other students' ethnoracial backgrounds. In response, 45 per cent said that it was "irrelevant," and 32 per cent said that it matters "somewhat," but they were "most interested in" the quality of the teaching and in the respect that people had for the related traditions, philosophies, and language. Only 20 per cent said that these issues mattered a great deal and that they would like to see more diversity, and only 3 per cent said that these issues both mattered a great deal and that they may leave their community if things do not improve.

58 Foxen, *Inhaling Spirit*.

59 Murphy, dir., *Eat, Pray, Love*.

Conclusion

1 Nin, *Seduction of the Minotaur*, 124. As Sady Doyle states in a sensitive account of the ways that the scandal-plagued Nin has re-emerged in the social media era, "she wrote for a world that did not yet exist, and so helped to bring it into being." Doyle, "Before Lena Dunham."

2 In the book's afterword, I reflect on issues that might be taken up by others in the future.

3 Altglas, *From Yoga to Kabbalah.*

4 Michael Adams and Andrew Parkin write, "Political leaders in Canada benefit from our inevitable tendency to compare ourselves to the United States. No matter how bad things are here, there is a good chance they are worse there. We have had fewer COVID deaths per capita, many fewer murders and mass shootings, and infinitely fewer losing politicians unwilling to accept voters' verdicts. Our health-care system is under tremendous strain, but there are still no fees for service." Adams and Parkin, "Differences between Canada."

5 This figure breaks down as follows: 43.4 per cent said that it was spiritual every time, 37.4 per cent said that it was spiritual sometimes, and 12 per cent said that it was spiritual "not often," which is a less enthusiastic way to say that it is at least sometimes spiritual. Our sample of 650 cannot be considered representative, of course. Nonetheless, the general trends that we see in this sample – regarding rates of practice, gender identity, socio-economic status, and approaches to health care – approximate other studies, our general expectations, and our experiences in the field. The rate of people indicating that yoga is a spiritual activity for them in this study, at 92.8 per cent, can be contrasted with what we found in the more representative sample of British Columbians sampled in the 2017 Pacific Northwest Social Survey, where 55 per cent of yoga practitioners in British Columbia reported that yoga was spiritual for them. Bramadat et al., eds, *Urban Religious Events*, 84. Given the decline in conventional religious practice and identification that we see throughout North America – with some exceptions to be found among evangelical Christians and immigration-driven newcomer communities – these are significant figures.

6 To put it in scholarly terms, "authorizing discourses" help to create a world with a particular arrangement of vested economic, political, gender, and professional interests. There is no way to escape authorizing discourses, but one can adopt more or less ironic approaches to the discourses in which one participates.

7 Letter of 9 February 1909, quoted in Swatos Jr, Kivisto, and Gustafson, "Weber, Max," 548.

8 Although I heard this saying first in a BBC documentary in 2023 about precarious citizenship among migrant workers in the United States, I have heard versions of it in yogaland and universityland.

9 Smith, *Soul Searching*. See also Watts, *Spiritual Turn*.

10 Van der Kolk, *Body Keeps the Score*.

11 I did not formally ask practitioners to reflect on yoga as a specific response to the current or impending climate catastrophes, although these matters did arise organically in many conversations in this study. Indeed, they have arisen many times during my decade in yogaland. Moreover, this speculation is consistent with a recent scholarly study whose authors found that "long-term yoga practice may create the internal conditions that make coping, mitigation, and adaptation somewhat easier and more desirable, potentially enhancing individual mental health, collective response capacity, and care for the planet." David, Buchan, and Nalau, "Coping and Adapting."

12 A senior teacher in Indianapolis noted, "[I was talking with a student] yesterday about how she loves [yoga], how yoga allows her to enter into a spiritual place through her body … It's such a dynamic, physical experience to go beyond our bodies. You know, what a paradox, right? The body's such a, a tool, a vehicle to go beyond it."

13 The last two items in this list deserve more attention than I have been able to offer in this book. On the first point, I note simply that yoga teaching as a career is often quite economically tenuous. North American teachers are paid in a variety of ways: per student, per hour, per class, in exchange for waiving the teacher's studio membership fees, or some combination of these. In 2023, the International Sports Sciences Association reported that full-time yoga instructors in the United States earn between roughly $45,000 and $75,000, with hourly rates ranging from $19 to $30. International Sports Sciences Association, "Yoga Instructor Salary." The salary range seems high to me. Even if we imagine that a teacher makes $100 per class, which would be quite a high average, and teaches two classes every day for five days of the week, with two weeks of holidays, their gross annual pay would be about $50,000. It is often the case that instructors need to work at several studios and in private homes; as well, in the United States, most teachers have to pay for their own health insurance. On the issue of conspirituality, see Ward and Voas, "Emergence of Conspirituality"; and Greenspan and Landsverk, "How QAnon Infiltrated."

14 Oliver, "Wild Geese," 347.

15 Marx, *Critique of Hegel's "Philosophy of Right,"* 131.

16 See respectively https://kinoyoga.com/; and https://yogawithadriene.com/.

17 Lucia, "Marking Sacred Space," 122.

18 The metaphor at work here – folding – was introduced in a compelling

keynote lecture by the American anthropologist Robert Weller at the International Society for the Sociology of Religion Conference, Taipei, Taiwan, 4–7 July 2023.

Afterword

1 In one community, a debate did emerge when a group of older cisgender feminist students learned that some people who were AMAB (assigned male at birth) trans women would be using the same change room as the AFAB (assigned female at birth) cisgender students. This debate was tumultuous, but the studio owner worked hard to keep her community together and lines of communication open. The concern was not about whether the studio should welcome trans people but about how the senior feminist students' concerns about change room etiquette might be addressed.

2 As a thought experiment, I randomly chose a province, a sphere of employment, and trans inclusion. My hunch was right, and LGBTQIA+ inclusion was built into the way that this Nova Scotian institution articulates itself to outsiders and insiders. See Government of Nova Scotia, *Guidelines to Support Trans*; and Nova Scotia Human Rights Commission, "June Is Pride Month."

3 For example, see Chaignon, "Yoga beyond the Binary."

4 The 2015 report of Truth and Reconciliation Commission of Canada and the commission's public hearings are sometimes mentioned as the culmination of these movements, but in fact they represent two milestones.

5 There were two notable exceptions to this pattern. One was a teacher in Vancouver who mentioned her Indigenous heritage, and the other was a teacher in Toronto who did not have Indigenous roots but included a territorial acknowledgment in her classes.

6 There were exceptions to this general trend too. One teacher in Indianapolis and five in New York were African American and spoke (if only briefly) about Black Lives Matter in their cities. They noted that they hoped that their presence and teaching style would broaden the appeal of yoga to other African Americans.

7 See, for example, Yoga Alliance, "Taking Action"; and IYNAUS, *Ethical Guidelines*.

8 Readers might recall Toni from chapter 1, where she said that she chose not to mix her politics with her yoga. Above, she frames the scandals as precursors of a spiritual revolution. Some would argue that she is guilty of "spiritual bypassing," the tendency to frame everything in spiritual terms in order to avoid difficult emotions or political problems. Arguably, this tendency is inherently

political in that it diverts attention from the more obvious causes of this misconduct (e.g., male privilege in this case).

9 Thom, "trauma is not sacred."

10 Laméris, "Bonfire Opera."

11 Iyengar, *Light on the Yoga Sutras*, 49.

12 Ibid., 52.

Bibliography

Adams, Michael, and Andrew Parkin. "The Differences between Canada and the US Remain Significant." *Policy Options*, 20 December 2022. https://policy options.irpp.org/magazines/december-2022/the-differences-between-canada-and-the-u-s-remain-significant/.

Alter, Joseph S. "Sacrifice, the Body, and Yoga: Theoretical Entailments of Embodiment in Hathayoga." *Journal of South Asian Studies* 35, no. 2 (2012): 408–33.

– "Yoga and Physical Education: Swami Kuvalayananda's Nationalist Project." *Asian Medicine* 3, no. 1 (2007): 20–36.

– *Yoga in Modern India: The Body between Philosophy and Science*. Princeton, NJ: Princeton University Press, 2004.

Alter, Joseph S., and Debra Diamond. "Yoga, Bodybuilding, and Wrestling: Metaphysical Fitness." In *Yoga: The Art of Transformation*, 85–94. Washington, DC: Arthur M. Sackler Gallery, Smithsonian Institute, 2013.

Altglas, Véronique. *From Yoga to Kabbalah: Religious Exoticism and the Logics of Bricolage*. New York: Oxford University Press, 2014.

American Psychiatric Association. "Climate Change and Mental Health Connections." n.d. https://www.psychiatry.org/patients-families/climate-change-and-mental-health-connections.

Anderson, Benedict. *Imagined Communities: Reflections on the Origins of Nationalism*. New York: Verso, 1991.

Archibong, Belinda, Brahima Sangafowa Coulibaly, and Ngozi Okonjo-Iweala. "How Have the Washington Consensus Reforms Affected Economic Performance in Sub-Saharan Africa?" Brookings Institution, 19 February 2021. https://www.brookings.edu/articles/how-have-the-washington-consensus-reforms-affected-economic-performance-in-sub-saharan-africa/.

Asad, Talal. *Formations of the Secular: Christianity, Islam, Modernity*. Stanford, CA: Stanford University Press, 2003.

– *Genealogies of Religion: Discipline and Reasons of Power in Christianity and Islam.* Baltimore, MD: Johns Hopkins University Press, 1993.

Baudon, Pauline, and Liza Jachens. "A Scoping Review of Interventions for the Treatment of Eco-anxiety." *International Journal of Environmental Research and Public Health* 18, no. 18 (2021): art 9636, 1–18. https://www.mdpi.com/1660-4601/18/18/9636.

Bender, Courtney. *The New Metaphysicals: Spirituality and the American Religious Imagination.* Chicago: University of Chicago Press, 2010.

Berger, Peter, and Thomas Luckmann. *The Social Construction of Reality: A Treatise in the Sociology of Knowledge.* London: Anchor Books, 1966.

Berila, Beth, Melanie Klein, and Chelsea Jackson Roberts, eds. *Yoga, the Body, and Embodied Social Change: An Intersectional Feminist Analysis.* Lanham, MD: Lexington Books, 2016.

Beyer, Peter, and Rubina Ramji. *Growing Up Canadian: Muslims, Hindus, Buddhists.* Montreal and Kingston: McGill-Queen's University Press, 2013.

B.K.S. Iyengar Yoga. "How to Become a Certified Iyengar Yoga Teacher (for Those Residing Outside of India)?" n.d. https://bksiyengar.com/modules/teacher/certeach.htm.

Black, Shameem. *Flexible India: Yoga's Cultural and Political Tensions.* New York: Columbia University Press, 2023.

Bouillier, Véronique. *Monastic Wanderers: Nath Yogi Ascetics in Modern South Asia.* London: Routledge, 2018.

Bramadat, Paul. "A Bridge Too Far: Yoga, Spirituality, and Contested Space in the Pacific Northwest." *Religion, State and Society* 47, nos 4–5 (2019): 491–507.

– *The Church on the World's Turf: An Evangelical Christian Group at a Secular University.* Oxford: Oxford University Press, 2000.

Bramadat, Paul, Benjamin L. Berger, and Noni MacDonald. "COVID-19 Vaccine: Religion, Trust and Vaccine Acceptance." Royal Society of Canada, 5 February 2021. https://rsc-src.ca/en/voices/covid-19-vaccine-religion-trust-and-vaccine-acceptance.

Bramadat, Paul, Mar Griera, Julia Martinez-Ariño, and Marian Burchardt, eds. *Urban Religious Events: Public Spirituality in Contested Spaces.* London: Bloomsbury, 2021.

Bramadat, Paul, Patricia O'Connell Killen, and Sarah Wilkins-LaFlamme, eds. *Religion at the Edge: Nature, Spirituality, and Secularity in the Pacific Northwest.* Vancouver: UBC Press, 2022.

Broad, William J. *The Science of Yoga: The Risks and Rewards.* New York: Simon and Schuster, 2012.

Brown, Candy Gunther. *Debating Yoga and Mindfulness in Public Schools: Reforming Secular Education or Reestablishing Religion?* Chapel Hill, NC: University of North Carolina Press, 2019.

Brown, Wendy. *Undoing the Demos: Neoliberalism's Stealth Revolution.* Princeton, NJ: Princeton University Press, 2017.

Bryant, Edwin. *The Yoga Sutras of Patanjali.* New York: North Point, 2009.

Bucar, Liz. *Stealing My Religion: Not Just Any Cultural Appropriation.* Cambridge, MA: Harvard University Press, 2022.

Burke, Tarana. *Unbound: My Story of Liberation and the Birth of the Me Too Movement.* New York: Flatiron Books, 2021.

Centre for Addictions and Mental Health. "Trauma." n.d. https://www.camh.ca/en/health-info/mental-illness-and-addiction-index/trauma.

Chaignon, Laura. "Yoga beyond the Binary." *Omstars*, 15 June 2021. https://omstars.com/blog/culture/yoga-beyond-the-binary/.

Cherniak, David, dir. "Nirvana in Nova Scotia." CBC Television, *Man Alive*, season 5, episode 12, 26 September 1995.

Chutkan, Robynne. *The Microbiome Solution: A Radical New Way to Heal Your Body from the Inside Out.* New York: Penguin, 2016.

Cope, Stephen. *Yoga and the Quest for the True Self.* New York: Bantam, 1999.

Creel, Bee. "How Much Will You Spend on Yoga Pants?" *Yoga Journal*, 8 December 2021. https://www.yogajournal.com/lifestyle/fashion-beauty/yoga-gear/least-to-most-expensive-yoga-pants/.

Csordas, Thomas J., ed. *Transnational Transcendence: Essays on Religion and Globalization.* Berkeley: University of California Press, 2009.

David, Tricia, Jenna Buchan, and Johanna Nalau. "Coping and Adapting to Climate Change in Australia: Yoga Perspectives." *International Journal of Yoga Therapy* 32 (2022): 1–15.

Daly, Natasha. "Fake Animal News Abounds on Social Media as Coronavirus Upends Life." *National Geographic*, 20 March 2020. https://www.nationalgeographic.com/animals/article/coronavirus-pandemic-fake-animal-viral-social-media-posts.

De Michelis, Elizabeth. *A History of Modern Yoga: Patanjali and Western Esotericism.* London: A&C Black, 2005.

– "Modern Yoga: Transmission of Theory and Practice." PhD dissertation, University of Cambridge, 2001.

Doniger, Wendy. *The Hindus: An Alternative History.* New York: Penguin, 2009.

Doyle, Sady. "Before Lena Dunham, There Was Anaïs Nin – Now Patron Saint of Social Media." *Guardian* (London), 8 April 2015. https://www.theguardian.com/culture/2015/apr/07/anais-nin-author-social-media.

Epstein, Mark. *The Trauma of Everyday Life.* Carlsbad, CA: Hay House, 2014.

Foxen, Anya. *Biography of a Yogi: Paramahansa Yogananda and the Origins of Modern Yoga.* New York: Oxford University Press, 2017.

– *Inhaling Spirit: Harmonialism, Orientalism, and the Western Roots of Modern Yoga.* New York: Oxford University Press, 2020.

Foxen, Anya, and Christa Kuberry. *Is This Yoga? Concepts, Histories, and the Complexities of Modern Practice.* London: Routledge, 2021.

Frerichs, Sabine. "Karl Polanyi and the Law of Market Society." *Österreichische Zeitschrift für Soziologie* 44 (2019): 197–208.

Gaudiani, Jennifer. *Sick Enough: A Guide to the Medical Complications of Eating Disorders.* London: Routledge, 2019.

Gandhi, Shreena, and Lillie Wolff. "Yoga and the Roots of Cultural Appropriation." Kalamazoo College Praxis Center, 19 December 2017. Posted at Trauma Sensitive Yoga, 23 April 2021. https://www.traumasensitiveyoganederland.com/yoga-and-the-roots-of-cultural-appropriation/.

Gilbert, Elizabeth. *Eat, Pray, Love: One Woman's Search for Everything across Italy, India, and Indonesia.* New York: Penguin, 2006.

Gleig, Ann. "The Culture of Narcissism Revisited: Transformations of Narcissism in Contemporary Psychospirituality." *Pastoral Psychology* 59, no. 1 (2010): 79–91.

Gleig, Ann, and Lola Williamson, eds. *Homegrown Gurus: From Hinduism in America to American Hinduism.* Albany: SUNY Press, 2013.

Godrej, Farah. "The Neoliberal Yogi and the Politics of Yoga. *Political Theory* 45, no. 6 (2017): 772–800.

Goldberg, Elliott. *The Path of Modern Yoga: The History of an Embodied Spiritual Practice.* Rochester, VT: Inner Traditions, 2016.

Government of India. *Common Yoga Protocol.* 2015. https://www.nacin.gov.in/resources/file/downloads/Common%20Yoga%20Protocol.pdf.

– "An Overview of the Department of AYUSH." n.d. https://ayush.gov.in/images/rti/rti6.pdf.

Government of Nova Scotia. *Guidelines to Support Trans and Gender Variant Employees.* n.d. https://beta.novascotia.ca/documents/how-support-trans-and-gender-variant-government-employees.

Greenspan, Rachel, and Daphne Landsverk. "How QAnon Infiltrated the Yoga World." *Business Insider*, 11 November 2020. https://www.businessinsider.com/qanon-conspiracy-theory-yoga-influencer-took-over-world-2020-11.

Griera, Mar. "Yoga in Penitentiary Settings: Transcendence, Spirituality, and Self-Improvement." *Human Studies* 40 (2017): 77–100.

Grigoriadis, Vanessa. "Karma Crash." *New York Magazine*, 13 April 2012. https://nymag.com/news/features/john-friend-yoga-2012-4/.

Griswold, Eliza. "Yoga Reconsiders the Role of the Guru in the Age of #MeToo." *New Yorker Magazine*, 23 July 2019. https://www.newyorker.com/news/news-desk/yoga-reconsiders-the-role-of-the-guru-in-the-age-of-metoo.

Guest, Matthew. *Neoliberal Religion: Faith and Power in the 21st Century*. London: Bloomsbury, 2022.

Hackett, Paul, ed. *The Assimilation of Yogic Religions through Pop Culture*. Lanham, MD: Rowman and Littlefield, 2017.

Halbfass, Wilhelm. *India and Europe: An Essay in Understanding*. Albany: SUNY Press, 1988.

Hall, David, ed. *Lived Religion in America: Toward a History of Practice*. Princeton, NJ: Princeton University Press, 1997.

Hari, Johann. "The Opposite of Addiction Isn't Sobriety – It's Connection." *Guardian* (London), 12 April 2016. https://www.theguardian.com/books/2016/apr/12/johann-hari-chasing-the-scream-war-on-drugs.

Heelas, Paul, and Linda Woodhead. *The Spiritual Revolution: Why Religion Is Giving Way to Spirituality*. Oxford: Wiley-Blackwell, 2005.

Herman, Judith. *Trauma and Recovery: The Aftermath of Violence from Domestic Abuse to Political Terror*. New York: Basic Books, 1992.

Hertzog Young, Charlie. "Diagnosing Climate Disorder." *Ecologist*, 27 September 2021. https://theecologist.org/2021/sep/27/diagnosing-climate-disorder.

International Sports Sciences Association. "Yoga Instructor Salary: How Much Does a Yoga Teacher Make?" *ISSA Online*, 21 June 2023. https://yoga.issaonline.com/blog/post/yoga-instructor-salary-how-much-does-a-yoga-teacher-make.

Iyengar, B.K.S. *Light on the Yoga Sutras of Patanjali*. 1993. Reprint, London: Harper-Collins, 1996.

IYNAUS [Iyengar Yoga National Association of the United States]. *Ethical Guidelines to Prevent Verbal Abuse, Sexual Harassment, and Physical Abuse*. 2019. https://iynaus.org/ethical-guidelines-to-prevent-verbal-abuse-sexual-harassment-and-physical-abuse/.

IYNAUS [Iyengar Yoga National Association of the United States] Board of Directors. "MM Investigative Report and Summary." [2019]. https://iynaus.org/wp-content/uploads/2021/04/MM-Investigative-Report-and-Summary-1.pdf.

Jain, Andrea R. "Fox News Controversy on Yoga and White Supremacy Reveals Problem of Yoga Discussion." *Religion Dispatches*, 7 February 2018. https://religion

dispatches.org/fox-news-controversy-on-yoga-and-white-supremacy-reveals-problem-of-yoga-discussion/.

– "Muktananda: Entrepreneurial Godman, Tantric Hero." In *Gurus of Modern Yoga*, ed. Mark Singleton and Ellen Goldberg, 190–209. New York: Oxford University Press, 2014.

– "Neoliberal Yoga." In *Routledge Handbook of Yoga and Meditation Studies*, ed. Suzanne Newcombe and Karen O'Brien-Kop, 51–62. New York: Routledge, 2020.

– *Peace Love Yoga: The Politics of Global Spirituality*. New York: Oxford University Press, 2020.

– *Selling Yoga: From Counterculture to Pop Culture*. New York: Oxford University Press, 2014.

Jois, Sharath. "Sharath Jois on the Essence of the Opening Prayer." *Sonima*, 18 January 2018. https://www.sonima.com/yoga/opening-prayer/.

Jones, Tasmin. "Traumatized Subjects: Continental Philosophy of Religion and the Ethics of Alterity." *Journal of Religion* 94, no. 2 (2014): 143–60.

Jung, Dietrich, and Stephan Stetter, eds. *Modern Subjectivities in World Society: Global Structures and Local Practices*. London: Palgrave Studies in International Relations, 2019.

Kadetsky, Elizabeth. *First There Is a Mountain: A Yoga Romance*. New York: Little, Brown, and Company, 2004.

Kale, Sunila S., and Christian Lee Novetzke. "The Cultural Politics of Yoga in India and the United States." In *At Home and Abroad: The Politics of American Religion*, ed. Elizabeth Shakman Hurd and Winnifred Fallers Sullivan, 210–27. New York: Columbia University Press, 2021.

Khoury, Nayla M., Jacqueline Lutz, and Zev Schuman-Olivier. "Interoception in Psychiatric Disorders: A Review of Randomized, Controlled Trials with Interoception-Based Interventions." *Harvard Review of Psychiatry* 26, no. 5 (2018): 250–63.

Korzybski, Alfred. "A Non-Aristotelian System and Its Necessity for Rigour in Mathematics and Physics." Paper presented at a meeting of the American Association for the Advancement of Science, New Orleans, Louisiana, 28 December 1931. http://esgs.free.fr/uk/art/sands-sup3.pdf.

Krishnamacharya, Sri Tirumulai. *Yoga Makaranda*. Trans. Lakshmi Ranganathan and Nandini Ranganathan. Madurai, India: CMV Press, 2006.

Lal, Neeta. "The Politics of Yoga: India's PM Has Been Aggressively Promoting the Practice. Not Everybody Is Happy about It." *Diplomat*, 4 April 2016. https://thediplomat.com/2016/04/the-politics-of-yoga/.

Laméris, Danusha. "Bonfire Opera." In *Bonfire Opera: Poems*. Pittsburgh, PA: University of Pittsburgh Press, 2020.

Lannert, Brittany K. "Traumatogenic Processes and Pathways to Mental Health Outcomes for Sexual Minorities Exposed to Bias Crime Information." *Trauma, Violence and Abuse* 16, no. 3 (2015): 291–8.

Lau, Lisa. "Re-Orientalism: The Perpetration and Development of Orientalism by Orientals." *Modern Asian Studies* 43, no. 2 (2009): 571–90.

Lau, Lisa, and Ana Mendes. *Re-Orientalism and South Asian Identity Politics: The Oriental Other Within*. London: Routledge, 2011.

Lavan, Spencer. *Unitarians and India: A Study in Encounter and Response*. 2nd ed. Boston: Skinner House, 1984.

Lessing, Doris. "Prisons We Choose to Live Inside – Part 1." Radio lecture, 29:36 mins. CBC *Massey Lectures*, 6 November 1985. https://www.cbc.ca/radio/ideas/the-1985-cbc-massey-lectures-prisons-we-choose-to-live-inside-1.2946839.

Lifestyle Desk. "International Yoga Day: 5 Yoga Gurus Who Were Accused of Sexual Assault." *Indian Express*, 21 June 2018. https://indianexpress.com/article/lifestyle/life-style/international-yoga-day-yoga-gurus-who-were-accused-of-sexual-assault-5226474/.

Lincoln, Bruce. *Holy Terrors: Thinking about Religion after September 11*. 2nd ed. Chicago: University of Chicago Press, 2006.

Lore, Benjamin. *Hell-Bent: Obsession, Pain, and the Search for Something Like Transcendence in Competitive Yoga*. New York: St Martin's Press, 2012.

Lucia, Amanda. "Guru Sex: Charisma, Proxemic Desire, and the Haptic Logics of the Guru-Disciple Relationship." *Journal of the American Academy of Religion* 86, no. 4 (2018): 953–88.

– "Marking Sacred Space: Altars and Yoga Mats in Transformative Events." *Journal of Festive Studies* 5 (2023): 110–30.

– *White Utopias: The Religious Exoticism of Transformational Festivals*. Berkeley: University of California Press, 2020.

Lukose, Ritty. "Decolonizing Feminism in the #MeToo Era." *Cambridge Journal of Anthropology* 36, no. 2 (2018): 34–52.

Macdonald, Helen. "Animals Are Rewilding Our Cities. On YouTube, at Least." *New York Times Magazine*, 15 April 2020. https://www.nytimes.com/2020/04/15/magazine/quarantine-animal-videos-coronavirus.html.

Maddeaux, Sabrina. "Yes, Overturning Roe v. Wade Affects Canadian Women." *National Post*, 28 June 2022. https://nationalpost.com/opinion/sabrina-maddeaux-yes-overturning-roe-v-wade-affects-canadian-women.

Maehle, Gregor. "Response to John Scott's View of Pattabhi Jois's Sexual Abuse by Karen Rain and Gregor Maehle." Chintamani Yoga, 9 October 2019. https://chintamaniyoga.com/response-to-john-scotts-view-of-pattabhi-joiss-sexual-abuse-by-karen-rain-and-gregor-maehle/.

– "My Initial Response to Karen Rain's Interview about Sexual Abuse." Chintamani Yoga, 17 May 2018. https://chintamaniyoga.com/my-initial-response-to-karen-rains-interview-about-sexual-abuse/.

Mallinson, James, and Mark Singleton. *Roots of Yoga*. London: Penguin Classics, 2017.

Martin, Craig. "Theses on the Critique of 'Religion.'" *Critical Research on Religion* 3, no. 1 (2015): 297–302.

Marx, Karl. *Critique of Hegel's "Philosophy of Right."* 1844. Trans. Annette Jolin and Joseph O'Malley. Cambridge, UK: Cambridge University Press, 1970.

Maté, Gabor. *In the Realm of Hungry Ghosts: Close Encounters with Addiction*. Toronto: Knopf Canada, 2008.

– *The Myth of Normal: Trauma, Illness, and Healing in a Toxic Culture*. Toronto: Knopf Canada, 2022.

McCartney, Patrick. "India's Battle against Egypt's Kimetic Yoga." *Medium*, 5 October 2021. https://psdmccartney.medium.com/indias-battle-against-egypt-s-kemetic-yoga-6eca5b114d65.

– "Politics beyond the Yoga Mat: Yoga Fundamentalism and the 'Vedic Way of Life.'" *Global Ethnographic* 4 (2017): 1–18.

– "Spiritual Bypass and Entanglement in Yogaland: How Neoliberalism, Soft Hindutva, and Banal Nationalism Facilitate Yoga Fundamentalism." *Politics and Religion Journal* 13, no. 1 (2019): 137–75.

McCutcheon, Russell. "A Default of Critical Intelligence? The Scholar of Religion as Public Intellectual." *Journal of the American Academy of Religion* 65, no. 2 (1997): 443–68.

McGowan, Victoria, and Clare Bambra. "COVID-19 Mortality and Deprivation: Pandemic, Syndemic, and Endemic Health Inequalities." *Lancet* 7, no. 11 (2022): E966–75.

McGuire, Meredith. *Lived Religion: Faith and Practice in Everyday Life*. New York: Oxford University Press, 2008.

Medin, R. Alexander, dir. *Mysore Magic: Yoga at the Source*. Documentary, 22 mins. Patanjali Productions and Upward Spiral Films, 2012.

Miller, Christopher Jain. *Embodying Transnational Yoga: Eating, Breathing, and Singing in Transformation*. London: Routledge, 2024.

Murphy, Ryan, dir. *Eat, Pray, Love*. Columbia Pictures, 2010.

Neumark-Sztainer, Dianne, Marla E. Eisenberg, Melanie Wall, and Katie A. Loth. "Yoga and Pilates: Associations with Body Image and Disordered Eating Behaviors in a Population-Based Sample of Young Adults." *International Journal of Eating Disorders* 44, no. 3 (2011): 276–80.

Nikias, Maria. "Yoga Lawsuit: Encinitas Union School District in California Sued over Classes." *ABC News*, 21 February 2013. https://abcnews.go.com/US/yoga-lawsuit-encinitas-union-school-district-california-sued/story?id=18561237.

Nin, Anaïs. *Seduction of the Minotaur*. 1961. Reprint, Chicago: Swallow, 1969.

Nova Scotia Human Rights Commission. "June Is Pride Month." 29 May 2023. https://humanrights.novascotia.ca/news-events/news/2023/june-pride-month.

Oliver, Mary. "Wild Geese." In *Devotions: The Collected Poems of Mary Oliver*, 347. New York: Penguin, 2017.

Orner, Eva, dir. *Bikram: Yogi, Guru, Predator*. Documentary, 86 mins. Pulse Films, 2019.

Pandell, Lexi. "How Trauma Became the Word of the Decade." *Vox*, 25 January 2022. https://www.vox.com/the-highlight/22876522/trauma-covid-word-origin-mental-health.

Perry, Tony. "Legal Fight against Yoga in Encinitas Schools Is Finished." *LA Times*, 12 June 2015. https://www.latimes.com/local/lanow/la-me-ln-yoga-legal-fight-20150612-story.html.

Pew Research Center. "Population Growth and Religious Composition." 21 September 2021. https://www.pewresearch.org/religion/2021/09/21/population-growth-and-religious-composition/.

Physiopedia. "Proprioception." n.d. https://www.physio-pedia.com/Proprioception.

Putnam, Robert. *Bowling Alone: The Collapse and Revival of American Community*. New York, Simon and Schuster 2000.

Rain, Karen. "Yoga Guru Pattabhi Jois Sexually Assaulted Me for Years." *Medium*, 9 October 2018. https://gen.medium.com/yoga-guru-pattabhi-jois-sexually-assaulted-me-for-years-48b3d04c9456.

Remski, Matthew. "How a #MeToo Facebook Post Toppled a Yoga Icon." *Medium*, 26 January 2020. https://gen.medium.com/how-a-metoo-facebook-post-toppled-a-yoga-icon-c25577185e40.

– "Shielded for Decades, a Yoga Leader's Alleged Sexual Abuse Finally Comes under Fire." *Medium*, 11 March 2020. https://gen.medium.com/shielded-for-decades-a-yoga-leaders-alleged-sexual-abuse-finally-comes-under-fire-97b79ddf990b.

– "Yoga's Culture of Sexual Abuse: Nine Women Tell Their Stories (Updated)." *Walrus*, 11 April 2023. https://thewalrus.ca/yogas-culture-of-sexual-abuse-nine-women-tell-their-stories/.

Riley, Angela R., and Kristen A. Carpenter. "Owning Red: A Theory of Indian (Cultural) Appropriation." *Texas Law Review* 94 (2015): 859–932.

Said, Edward. *Orientalism*. New York: Pantheon Books, 1978.

Sarbacker, Stuart Ray. *Tracing the Path of Yoga: The History and Philosophy of Indian Mind-Body Discipline*. Albany: SUNY Press, 2021.

Scheeringa, Michael. *The Trouble with Trauma: The Search to Discover How Beliefs Become Facts*. Las Vegas, NV: Central Recovery, 2021.

Schettler, Renee Marie. "He Faced Allegations of Sexual Assault and Rape from Students for Years. Now Bikram Choudhury Is 'Back' Teaching in Canada." *Yoga Journal*, 9 February 2023. https://www.yogajournal.com/lifestyle/bikram-choudhury-teaching-yoga/.

Scott, David. "The Rise of India: UK Perspectives." *International Affairs* 93, no. 1 (2017): 165–88.

Scott, John. "My Yoga Teacher: K. Pattabhi Jois – Guruji or Not, Enlightened or Not, Guru or Sexual Abuser." 23 August 2018. https://www.johnscottyoga.com/about/my-teacher/.

Sharath Yoga Centre. "Authorisation." 13 May 2022. https://sharathyogacentre.com/2022/05/13/authorisation/.

Shaw, Alison. "'A Tool to Help Me through the Darkness': Suffering and Healing among Teacher-Practitioners of Ashtanga Yoga." *Anthropology and Medicine* 28 (2021): 320–40.

Shearer, Alistair. *The Story of Yoga: From Ancient India to the Modern West*. London: Hurst and Company, 2020.

Sherov-Ignatiev, Vladimir G., and Sergei F. Sutyrin. "Peculiarities and Rationale of Asymmetric Regional Trade Agreements." World Trade Organization, n.d. https://www.wto.org/english/res_e/publications_e/wtr11_forum_e/wtr11_2aug11_a_e.htm.

Singleton, Mark. *Yoga Body: The Origins of Modern Posture Practice*. New York: Oxford University Press, 2010.

Singleton, Mark, and Ellen Goldberg, eds. *Gurus of Modern Yoga*. New York: Oxford University Press, 2014.

Sivananda. "Statement by the Board of Directors of the International Sivananda Yoga Vedanta Centres." 16 December 2019. https://web.archive.org/web/20191217211502/https://sivananda.org/.

Slatoff, Zoë. "Sacred Sound." Ashtanga Yoga Sanskrit, n.d. https://www.ashtangayo gasanskrit.com/yoga-sanskrit-and-philosophy-classes.

Smith, Christian. *Soul Searching: The Religious and Spiritual Lives of American Teenagers*. New York: Oxford University Press, 2005.

School of Oriental and African Studies, University of London. "The Hatha Yoga Project: Ancient Practices for Modern Wellbeing." n.d. https://www.soas.ac.uk/ research/hatha-yoga-project-ancient-practices-modern-wellbeing.

Stern, Eddie. *One Simple Thing: A New Look at the Science of Yoga and How It Can Transform Your Life*. New York: North Point, 2019.

Strauss, Sarah. *Positioning Yoga: Balancing Acts across Cultures*. Oxford: Berg, 2005.

Stringfellow, Susan. "The Politics of Yoga Pants." *Yoga International*, n.d. https:// yogainternational.com/article/view/the-politics-of-yoga-pants/.

Stukin, Stacie. "Yogi Bhajan Turned an L.A. Yoga Studio into a Juggernaut, and Left Two Generations of Followers Reeling from Alleged Abuse." *Los Angeles Magazine*, 15 July 2020. https://lamag.com/featured/yogi-bhajan.

Swatos, William H., Jr, Peter Kivisto, and Paul M. Gustafson. "Weber, Max." In *Encyclopedia of Religion and Society*, ed. William H. Swatos Jr, 547–52. Walnut Creek, CA: AltaMira, 1998. http://hirr.hartsem.edu/ency/Weber.htm.

Syman, Stefanie. *The Subtle Body: The Story of Yoga in America*. New York: Farrar, Straus and Giroux, 2010.

Thatamanil, John J. *Circling the Elephant: A Comparative Theology of Religious Diversity*. New York: Fordham University Press, 2020.

Thom, Kai Cheng. "trauma is not sacred." In *a place called No Homeland*. Vancouver: Arsenal Pulp, 2017. https://onbeing.org/poetry/trauma-is-not-sacred/.

van der Kolk, Bessel. *The Body Keeps the Score: Brain, Mind and Body in the Healing of Trauma*. New York: Viking, 2014.

van der Veer, Peter, and Steven Vertovec. "Brahmanism Abroad: On Caribbean Hinduism as an Ethnic Religion." *Ethnology* 30, no. 2 (1991): 149–66.

Vanzee Taylor, Laura, dir. *I am Maris: Portrait of a Young Yogi*. Documentary, 54 mins. ro*co films, 2018. https://www.iammarismovie.com/.

Vishuddhi Films. "Yogacharya BKS Iyengar's Unique Revelations." Video, 14:36 mins. *YouTube*, 30 November 2015. Excerpt from the documentary *History of Yoga: The Path of My Ancestors*, dir. Deepika Kothari and Ramji Om, 1 hr, 38 mins. Vishuddhi Films, 2015. https://www.youtube.com/watch?v=ogHioB8_gFU.

Vitello, Paul. "Hindu Group Stirs a Debate over Yoga's Soul." *New York Times*, 27 November 2010. https://www.nytimes.com/2010/11/28/nyregion/28yoga.html.

Wallace, Benjamin. "Bikram Feels the Heat." *Vanity Fair*, January 2014. https://archive.vanityfair.com/article/2014/1/bikram-feels-the-heat.

Wallace, David Foster. *Infinite Jest*. New York: Little, Brown, and Company 1996.

Ward, Charlotte, and David Voas. "The Emergence of Conspirituality." *Journal of Contemporary Religion* 26, no. 1 (2011): 103–21.

Watts, Galen. *The Spiritual Turn: The Religion of the Heart and the Making of Romantic Liberal Modernity*. New York: Oxford University Press, 2022.

White, David Gordon. *Sinister Yogis*. Chicago: University of Chicago Press, 2010.

– *The Yoga Sutra of Patanjali: A Biography*. Princeton, NJ: Princeton University Press, 2014.

– ed. *Yoga in Practice*. Princeton, NJ: Princeton University Press, 2011.

Wildcroft, Theodora. *Post-lineage Yoga: From Guru to #MeToo*. London: Equinox, 2020.

Wittich, Agi, and Patrick McCartney. "Changing Face of the Yoga Industry, Its Dharmic Roots and Its Message to Women: An Analysis of Yoga Journal Magazine Covers, 1975–2020." *Journal of Dharma Studies* 3, no. 1 (2020): 31–44.

Wolf, Naomi. *The Beauty Myth: How Images of Beauty Are Used against Women*. New York: William Morrow, 1991.

Woodhead, Linda, and Andrew Brown. *That Was the Church That Was: How the Church of England Lost the English People*. London: Bloomsbury, 2016.

YJ Editors. "Kausthub Desikachar Faces Abuse Allegations." *Yoga Journal*, 27 September 2021. https://www.yogajournal.com/lifestyle/kausthub-desikachar-faces-abuse-allegations/.

Yoga Alliance. "About Us: Our Story." n.d. https://yogaalliance.org/about-us/.

– "RYS 200 Standards." n.d. https://www.yogaalliance.org/credentialing/standards/200-hourstandards.

– "Sexual Misconduct Policy." February 2020. https://www.yogaalliance.org/About_Us/Policies/Policy_Prohibiting_Sexual_Misconduct.

– "Taking Action against Sexual Misconduct." n.d. https://www.yogaalliance.org/Portals/0/Articles/Sexual_Misconduct_Action_YA.pdf?ver=2020-01-06-144944-070.

– "The Yoga Diversity Dilemma." 12 July 2016. https://www.yogaalliance.org/About_Yoga/Article_Archive/The_Yoga_Diversity_Dilemma.

– *Yoga in the World*. 2023. https://www.yogaalliance.org/yoga_in_the_world.

Yoga Journal Staff. "#TimesUp: Ending Sexual Abuse in the Yoga Community." *Yoga Journal*, 12 February 2018. https://www.yogajournal.com/lifestyle/balance/sex/timesup-metoo-ending-sexual-abuse-in-the-yoga-community.

Yogananda, Paramahansa. *Autobiography of a Yogi*. 1946. Reprint, Los Angeles, CA: Self-Realization Fellowship, 1998.

Index